midnight
meditations

calm your thoughts, still your body,
and return to sleep

courtney e. ackerman

ADAMS MEDIA

NEW YORK LONDON TORONTO SYDNEY NEW DELHI

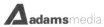

Adams Media
An Imprint of Simon & Schuster, Inc.
100 Technology Center Drive
Stoughton, Massachusetts 02072

First Adams Media hardcover edition
June 2021

ADAMS MEDIA and colophon are
trademarks of Simon & Schuster.

For information about special discounts for
bulk purchases, please contact Simon &
Schuster Special Sales at 1-866-506-1949
or business@simonandschuster.com.

The Simon & Schuster Speakers Bureau
can bring authors to your
live event. For more information
or to book an event contact the Simon &
Schuster Speakers Bureau
at 1-866-248-3049 or visit our website
at www.simonspeakers.com.

Interior design by Julia Jacintho
Illustrations by Emma Taylor

Manufactured in the
United States of America

1 2021

Library of Congress Cataloging-in-
Publication Data
Names: Ackerman, Courtney E., author.
Title: Midnight meditations / Courtney
E. Ackerman.
Description: First Adams Media
hardcover edition. | Stoughton,
Massachusetts: Adams Media, 2021. |
Identifiers: LCCN 2021000301 |
ISBN 9781507216064 (hc) | ISBN
9781507216071 (ebook)
Subjects: LCSH: Meditation. |
Meditations. | Sleep.
Classification: LCC BF637.M4 A25
2021 | DDC 158.1/28--dc23
LC record available at
https://lccn.loc.gov/2021000301

ISBN 978-1-5072-1606-4
ISBN 978-1-5072-1607-1 (ebook)

contents

chapter one
breath meditations ... 17

chapter two
body meditations ... 49

chapter three
thought meditations ... 81

chapter four
emotion meditations ... 113

chapter five

visualization meditations ... 145

introduction

We've all been there—suddenly awake in the middle of the night, tossing and turning, with our minds racing. We wake up for a variety of reasons, from simply falling asleep in an uncomfortable position to a problem weighing heavily on our minds. Whatever the reason, it's frustrating to find yourself alert and awake when all you want is a little rest.

It's a common problem, but the good news is that you don't have to sit and stew while you wait for sleep to overtake you again. Calming meditations like the 150 options in this book can help your mind and body relax and get you back to sleep in no time. *Midnight Meditations* offers several techniques designed to lead you back into dreamland: breathing exercises, visualizations, body-focused meditations, and more. You might find that one technique is more effective for you than others, or you might find that certain methods work better in specific situations. For example, breathing exercises might help when you're stressed, while body-focused meditations may be most effective when your body is stiff or sore. You can read through all the meditations in this book first, or feel free to jump right to one that resonates with you (they are organized by technique). Different meditations will hit the spot at different times, so make sure to try lots of the many options.

Above all, try not to get too frustrated or anxious when you wake up unexpectedly. The best way to fall back asleep is to forget that you "should" be asleep right now. The more you focus on what you "should" be doing, the harder it is to relax enough to actually do it. The meditations in this book use a variety of methods to help you get back to sleep, but they all start with soothing your busy brain to a relaxed state and giving it permission to shut off again. That's the key to getting back to sleep.

So, while you flip through this book to find a meditation that you think might work for you, remember to show yourself some compassion and go easy on your busy, all-too-alert brain. We rarely get back to sleep by berating ourselves or thinking of all the things that annoy us, so skip that approach and get right to the ones that work.

Let these meditations help you lie back, let go, and drift into peaceful slumber once again. Give your overworked body and mind the restful and restorative time they deserve—each and every night.

how to use this book

This book provides 150 different meditations for you to use when you wake up in the night and want to get right back to sleep. There are meditations in a variety of techniques for you to choose from, so you're sure to find one that works for you no matter how alert you are when you first open this book.

To maximize the effectiveness of these meditations, I'd like to offer some suggestions on how to use them. Before practicing any sort of meditation, pause, take a moment to focus on yourself and how you are feeling, and cultivate some mindfulness. Mindfulness is all about being aware of yourself and being present in the current moment. Meditation and mindfulness go hand in hand, and it's a great idea to gear yourself up for meditation by being more mindful.

It's also a good idea to set an intention before you meditate. For a general meditation, ask yourself what you would like to do during this time you're carving out just for you. What do you hope to get from this experience? How would you like to feel afterward? Of course, if you're using *this* book, your intention is to get back to sleep. But you may want to set other, more specific, intentions before engaging in any of these meditations, like "My intention is to relax and ease the tension in my shoulders" or "My intention is to let go of this thought that's been bothering me." Your intention will help guide your meditation practice and keep you on track.

You can meditate in any position or posture you like, but there are two postures that are most often adopted when meditating: sitting upright (either in a chair or on the floor/a cushion with crossed legs) or lying flat on your back. Lying flat on your back will probably help you get back to sleep more quickly than sitting upright; however, it's up to you how you want to meditate. In some cases, you might feel more comfortable sitting than lying down. Unless otherwise noted in the meditation, you can choose whichever position feels better in the moment.

Likewise, you have two options for your eyes: You can leave them open with a soft focus (i.e., glazed eyes, looking at nothing in particular), or you can keep them gently closed (not squeezed shut). Closed eyes will likely get you back to a sleepy state better than open eyes, but you may find that's not the case for you. Feel free to give both a try and see what works. Unless otherwise noted in the meditation, you can go with either option.

Posture and eyelid position can affect your results, but the most important things you can do to prepare for these meditations are to:

1. Acknowledge that you are currently awake when you'd rather be asleep, but accept that this is the way it is.

2. Decide to be open to whichever exercise you choose.

3. Follow the instructions and give it a chance to work.

Happy meditating!

chapter one

breath meditations

come back to your breath

This meditation is a building block of a good meditation practice. It focuses on your breath and is very simple, as there is only one rule: Come back to your breath. Follow these instructions to give it a try:

1. **You can be either seated or lying down for this exercise—just make sure you feel comfortable and can breathe easily.**

2. **Focus on your breath. Think about how it feels to breathe. Notice how you draw in and then expel air.**

3. **Eventually, you will not be able to focus solely on your breath anymore, and your mind will wander. Don't beat yourself up about this; it's a common occurrence in meditation. When you catch your mind wandering, simply bring it back to your breath. Do so gently, and with compassion for your busy mind.**

4. **Continue focusing on your breath and bringing your mind back to it when it wanders.**

If you feel you've been focusing on your breath for a while and you are still not sleepy, try setting a timer with a soft, soothing sound for 5 minutes. If you don't feel sleepy after 5 minutes of focusing on your breath, try a different meditation.

breathe in a square

Focusing on your breath is a simple way to gently lull your busy mind back to sleep. There are several effective techniques, including this "square" breathing method. With this exercise, focus all your attention on your breath as you purposefully breathe in, breathe out, and take meaningful pauses. With this method, you spend equal amounts of time breathing in, holding your breath in, breathing out, and then pausing. This creates four equal "sides" to your breath, making a square. The square breathing method ensures that you take in enough oxygen during your in-breaths and challenges your lungs when holding between in- and out-breaths. In addition to being good for your lungs, this technique helps settle and clear your mind, giving you the peace you need to drift back to sleep. Here's how it works:

1. **Gently breathe in through your nose for 4 seconds.**
2. **Hold your breath for 4 seconds.**
3. **Gently exhale through your nose for 4 seconds.**
4. **Pause for 4 seconds.**
5. **Repeat steps 1 through 4 at least 5 times.**

If you find yourself still struggling to get back to sleep, repeat the exercise or try the "difficult mode" version: breathe in, hold, breathe out, and pause for 5 seconds each.

try full-capacity breathing

How often do you breathe at full capacity? Probably not that often. This exercise is easy because sometimes all you need is a simple reminder to breathe fully in order to relax and get back to sleep. Give this exercise a try to promote relaxation and calm:

1. **Breathe in deeply through your nose until your lungs are completely full. Breathe in a little longer than you think you need to.**

2. **Pause for just a moment when your lungs are full.**

3. **Breathe out deeply through your nose until your lungs are completely empty. Again, go a little longer than you think is necessary.**

4. **Repeat at least 5 times.**

It's important to push yourself a little farther than you normally do when filling and emptying your lungs. It might feel a little uncomfortable, but it's worth it. Your lung capacity is far larger than you think it is, and your brain just needs a reminder of how much you can take in and push out.

We naturally tend toward shallow breaths—especially when we're stressed—but using your full capacity to breathe will put your brain in a more relaxed and calm state and make it easier for you to fall asleep.

watch your breath

There are many exercises based on changing your breathing that can help induce calm and make it easier to fall asleep, but simply paying attention to your breath can do the same thing. Try just following your breath instead of changing it. Here's how you do it:

1. **Get extra-comfy in a position that makes it easy to breathe.**

2. **With your eyes open, turn your eyes to your chest and turn your attention to your breath.**

3. **Approach your breath with fascination, feeling the air enter and exit your lungs as your body moves with the breath. Note how it feels to breathe in and breathe out as you watch your chest rise and fall.**

4. **Continue to follow your breath wherever it goes for at least 10 breaths.**

This exercise instructs you to watch your breath—that's it. Seeing your torso move as the air travels in and out of your lungs will ground you in the present moment, making it easier to switch off the errant thoughts and neutralize anxieties that seem so much more active at night.

Focus all of your attention on your breath and watch it with interest and curiosity to soothe your mind back to a sleepy state.

feel each breath

How often do you really pay attention to how each breath feels? Focus on feeling each breath with these steps:

1. Take a deep breath in through your mouth, paying attention to how it feels when the air travels down your throat and into your lungs.

2. Release that deep breath, also through your mouth, and pay attention to the sensations you feel as the air travels back up from your lungs, through your throat, and out your mouth.

3. Now, take another deep breath, this time in through your nose. Focus on how it feels in your body to take in a breath this way.

4. Release your breath again, this time through your nose. Note the sensations in your chest and belly as you exhale.

5. Think about how it felt to breathe in through your mouth and through your nose, and note which was more relaxing. Continue breathing and paying close attention to the sensations you feel with each breath.

Even if you have paid attention to your breath before, you may not have focused on how it actually *feels*. Keeping your mind busy with the sensations you're experiencing will make it easier to feel calm and sleepy, gently lulling you back to dreamland.

direct your breath

If you are feeling tight, tense, or uncomfortable when you wake up, this is a good choice to help you fall back to sleep. You will direct your breath to wherever it needs to go to help you relax and de-stress. Follow these steps to direct your breath:

1. Think about what part of your body is feeling the tightest or most tense.

2. Breathe in deeply through your nose, feeling your breath as it travels into your nostrils and down to your lungs.

3. Breathe out fully, mindful of the sensations as your breath leaves your airway.

4. Now, think of the spot that is feeling tight or tense. For your next in-breath, focus on that spot and imagine sending your breath directly to it. Follow your breath in your mind as it travels to that spot in your body. See it permeate this spot in your body.

5. As you breathe out, watch your breath leave this spot and travel out through your nostrils.

6. Continue breathing this way, directing your breath to and from the tense spot in your body, for at least 10 breaths.

It's often the shoulders or neck that hold tension when we're stressed, but any part of your body can be tight and tense, so pay close attention to how your body is feeling before you begin.

breathe in bursts

If you're feeling a little wound up or too energetic to get back to sleep, this exercise is the perfect one to try. You're going to use your breath to release that extra energy so you can slide back into a sleepy state. Here's how it works:

1. **Start with a slow, steady breath to focus on your breathing. Breathe deeply—in through your nose for 4 seconds and out through your nose for 4 seconds.**

2. **Now that your attention is focused on your breathing, switch to short bursts. Take your next breath in using 4 short, sharp bursts. In other words, use 4 in-breaths to fill up your lungs as quickly as you can. It should only take about a second.**

3. **Breathe out in short bursts as well, using 4 quick out-breaths to empty your lungs. This should also take only a second to do.**

4. **Continue this "in, in, in, in, out, out, out, out" pattern 20 times. Notice how you're feeling at the end. If you still feel full of energy, repeat the pattern 20 more times. Eventually, you will discharge all your excess energy and feel calmer and more relaxed.**

You can think of this exercise as getting rid of the static charge you sometimes get when you walk on carpet. You have to find someplace to release that energy, such as touching something metal, in order to rid yourself of it.

fill a breath balloon

This exercise combines a breathing technique with a bit of visualization to give you a calming method to relax and get back to a sleepy state of mind. Try filling a breath balloon to get your mind ready for slumber again. Here are the steps:

1. With your eyes closed, imagine that a balloon is fixed to your nose, covering both nostrils. If this idea makes you feel anxious, imagine it covers just one nostril instead. The balloon is about half full of air.

2. As you breathe in through your nose, watch as the balloon empties, giving you all the air inside of it.

3. As you breathe out through your nose, watch as the balloon fills, rising and expanding with the air from your lungs.

4. Keep this image in mind as you breathe steadily in and out for 10 breaths. Try to slow your breath a little bit each time, but also try to fill the balloon a little fuller each time. If you're still having trouble sleeping, try repeating this exercise for a longer period of time (e.g., 5 or 10 minutes).

This exercise gets your brain focused on your breath in a way that not only distracts it from the unfortunate fact that it's awake; it also provides a soothing, relaxing energy to lull it back to sleep. Filling the balloon gives your mind something to "do" while your body calms it with the breath.

float on your breath

If you have fond memories of floating on a lake, river, or pool, you'll love this exercise. It's designed to give you the same sense of peace and relaxation you get when you're floating on water without a care. Here's how to do it:

1. **Think of a time when you peacefully, joyfully floated on water. If you don't have any such memories to recall, imagine it instead. You're spread out on the water, with your face up to the warmth of the sun, body gently rocked by the waves.**

2. **While you float, match your breathing to the motion of your body. As you breathe in, feel your body rise slightly as if reaching the top of a small wave.**

3. **As you breathe out, feel your body fall as you reach the trough of that small wave.**

4. **Continue breathing full, deep breaths and matching your floating movements with them. Rise and fall gently, slowly, with each breath.**

Water is one of the most calming elements to add to your meditations. It has a soothing, healing quality that is deeply rooted in us, perhaps going back to when we floated safe and secure in the womb. Incorporating it into your meditations is an excellent way to induce calm and help you drift back to sleep.

breathe in calm, blow out tension

This meditation is a wonderful way to soothe your worried mind back to sleep if you're awake with tension or anxiety:

1. With your eyes either gently closed or open with a soft, relaxed focus, bring your attention to your breath.

2. Find a breathing rhythm that feels good for you, preferably one that's slow and steady. Continue breathing this way for a few breaths and get comfortable.

3. Now, imagine that all the tension, anxiety, and stress is sitting in your mind, coiled like a snake. It's a jumble of threads of all different colors.

4. As you breathe in, imagine a white mist of calm coming in through your nostrils and into your mind.

5. As you breathe out, imagine those threads untangling and exiting your mind through your nostrils.

6. With each breath, you breathe in that calm, soothing white mist and you breathe out a little more of those tension threads. Continue until all the threads have left your mind and only the white mist remains.

This meditation uses some visualization but still focuses on your breath as the primary method of removing tension and replacing it with calm. With each breath, you will slowly shift the balance of tension and calm in your mind, allowing you to drift back to sleep.

count your breaths

Just like counting sheep can help you get to sleep when you're feeling restless, counting your breaths can be a great way to soothe a busy mind. Try this meditation to get back to a sleepy state:

1. You can choose whether you want to sit or lie down for this exercise—pick whichever is more comfortable for you in this moment. You can also choose whether you want your eyes closed or open with a soft focus; one might be easier and more relaxing for you than the other.

2. Once you're settled and in a comfortable position, turn your full attention to your breath. Notice how it feels as your chest rises on an in-breath and falls on an out-breath.

3. Now, with your attention focused on your breath, start counting each breath. You can count as you breathe in, as you reach the top of the breath (with your lungs full), as you breathe out, or at the bottom of each breath (with your lungs empty); the choice is yours.

4. Continue counting each breath. If you lose track at some point, simply start back at 1 and continue on. Count up to 30 breaths.

Counting things is an old trick to calm your mind back to sleep, and adding a focus on your breath makes it even more effective. It allows your mind to take a break from worrying or ruminating and instead focuses your attention on the easy, calming task at hand.

challenge yourself with 6-second breathing

This is a more advanced breathing technique that is great for bringing a sense of peace to the mind; however, it may not be right for those with limited lung function. Give it a try to see if it will work for you. (If it doesn't, try the "Breathe in a Square" meditation instead.) Follow these instructions to try it out:

1. Take a slow, deep breath in, counting to 6 as you go. Try to breathe steadily, taking in air at the same rate throughout the in-breath.

2. Pause for a moment at the top of the breath (when your lungs are full).

3. Slowly release all the air in your lungs, again counting to 6 as you exhale. Breathe out steadily as well, expelling air at the same rate throughout the out-breath.

4. Pause again for a brief moment at the bottom of the breath (when your lungs are empty).

5. Repeat the 6-second breath 10 times.

This is an advanced technique but a simple exercise. All you need to do is breathe in deeply for 6 seconds and breathe out for another 6 seconds. If you have the lung capacity for it, this breathing technique will leave you feeling calm, serene, and ready to sleep.

try alternate nostril breathing

Alternate nostril breathing is a meditative practice that can fill a busy mind with feelings of calmness and serenity. It's easy to do once you get the hang of it. Here's how to try alternate nostril breathing to lull yourself back to sleep:

1. Take either hand and fold in all fingers but the pinkie and the thumb (making the "hang loose" sign with your hand).

2. Place your thumb on the right or left nostril (right nostril if you're using your right hand, left nostril if you're using your left hand). I'll use the right nostril first to explain the rest of the exercise.

3. With your right nostril closed, breathe in steadily through your left nostril.

4. Pause for a moment while you remove your thumb from your right nostril and place your pinkie over your left nostril.

5. With your left nostril closed, breathe out steadily through your right nostril.

6. Alternate back and forth, breathing in and out through one nostril, then the other. Repeat this for 10 breaths.

Alternate nostril breathing will distract your hyperactive mind and focus it on its task of switching the breath from one nostril to the other. If you're still awake and alert after 10 breaths, switch to a less dynamic breathing exercise.

create some wind

Sometimes what we need to fall asleep is a little whimsy. When we take things too seriously, we have trouble relaxing and letting go, and anxiety gets the better of us. Try this meditation practice to get silly instead of serious. Here's how to create some whimsical wind:

1. **With your eyes open and a soft focus, open your mouth and take in a deep breath, the deepest you've taken all day.**

2. **Hold your breath in for a moment.**

3. **Make your mouth into an "O" shape and let your breath out in one big, forceful exhale. Move your jaw and your lips to direct the "wind" different ways. Make it go left, right, up, down, in a circle, whatever feels fun to you.**

4. **Repeat these steps a few times, letting yourself get caught up in the fantasy. Can you make something flutter in the breeze across the room? See if you can send the "wind" all the way up to the ceiling.**

If you're feeling seriously frustrated at your lack of ability to fall back asleep, sometimes a more lighthearted exercise is just what you need. Lighten up, let go of tension, and create some wind to relax enough that you can get back to sleep.

be the fan

Smooth motion, repetition, and deep breathing—what do they all have in common? They can all help you get back to sleep. This technique employs all three to activate your sleep mode. To get yourself sleepy again, try these steps:

1. **Sit upright in a comfortable position. Even if you prefer to lie down to meditate, this exercise is best if you are seated.**

2. **Look straight ahead and close your eyes. As you breathe in, slowly turn your head to your right.**

3. **Pause for just a moment, then breathe out as you slowly move your head back to center.**

4. **Breathe in again as you turn your head to the left.**

5. **Pause for a moment again, then breathe out as you slowly move your head back to center.**

6. **This sequence represents 1 repetition. Do 10 repetitions to soothe your mind back to a sleepy state.**

There's a reason parents often rub their children's backs with long, soft strokes when they want them to go back to sleep; the smooth motions and repetition are relaxing and help us feel safe and comforted, which can get our mind and body in the right state to sleep. Add deep breathing, and you've got a recipe for sleep.

try constant breathing

This technique may help you release some pent-up tension and get safely back to sleep, or it may add a little energy to your mind and body. The result depends on how you normally breathe throughout the day and what associations you have with steady breathing; for example, martial artists and yogis may be energized, since it brings to mind their practice. If it gives you energy instead of making you tired, use a different exercise (and save this one for a time when you need to wake up!). These are the steps:

1. **In a comfortable position of your choice, take a moment to focus on your breath. Note when and where you pause before inhaling or exhaling, and for how long you pause. You're about to try to nix that pause.**

2. **Begin by breathing in slowly and steadily until your lungs are full.**

3. **As soon as your lungs are full, begin breathing out just as slowly and steadily until your lungs are empty.**

4. **Repeat steps 2 and 3 at least 10 times, constantly breathing throughout that time.**

Many—perhaps most—of the breathing techniques that can help you get back to sleep involve pausing between breaths. These pauses can be really effective, but this alternate method encourages you to engage in constant, seamless breathing, in which your breath is one long, continuous motion instead of several short motions back-to-back.

engage in ujjayi breathing

Ujjayi breath is a popular breathing exercise that has been used for hundreds, perhaps even thousands, of years. It is often done in yoga classes and meditation practices, and it can also help lull you to a peaceful sleep. Here's how ujjayi breathing works:

1. Sit tall, with the top of your head reaching up to the ceiling.

2. Make a soft restriction at the back of your throat, where your glottis is. This allows a little less air to pass through at a time and gives your breath the "Darth Vader" sound.

3. Breathe in slowly but naturally, inhaling as long as you'd like.

4. Pause for just a moment, then exhale the same way: slowly and steadily, and for the same amount of time.

5. Repeat steps 2 through 4 at least 10 times, listening for the rushing sound as you breathe in and out.

The ujjayi breath, also known as "ocean breath" for its distinctive sound, connects your belly, rib cage, chest, throat, and mouth in a harmonious and soothing breathing practice, helping you be present in your body and bring calm to your mind. Many yogis attempt to bring ujjayi breath to every yoga practice in order to stay calm and balanced.

employ 4-7-8 breathing

The 4-7-8 breathing method is a good choice for relaxing and letting go of stress and tension in the body and in the mind. It was discovered by Dr. Andrew Weil, an expert in integrative medicine. He found that it helped people take control of their body and mind through taking control of their breath, helping them lessen their anxiety and allowing them to relax enough to fall back to sleep. Follow these simple instructions to give it a try:

1. While seated or lying down, get comfortable and close your eyes and mouth.
2. Inhale quietly and steadily through your nose for 4 seconds.
3. With your lungs full of air, hold your breath in for 7 seconds.
4. Exhale quietly and steadily through your mouth for a total of 8 seconds, making a "whoosh" sound as you do.
5. Repeat the 4-7-8 cycle 10 times.

The in-breath through your nose helps your mind relax, while holding your breath for a prolonged period of time gives your lungs a chance to move all that oxygen to where it's needed throughout your body. Breathing out steadily helps your mind and body find balance again, which allows you to rest easy and relax back into sleep.

double your exhale

Breathing in and breathing out are both necessary, of course, but they trigger different emotional responses in the brain. Breathing in can be energizing and uplifting, and breathing out can be relaxing and relieving. Try focusing on your exhale to get more relaxed. Here's what to do:

1. **Get cozy and take a few deep breaths to get started. Keep your eyes open for now with a soft focus.**

2. **Now, take in a normal, natural-feeling inhale and count how many seconds it is. It's probably between 1 and 3 seconds, but it may be longer if you're relaxed.**

3. **Continue breathing at this rate, but make your exhale twice as long. For example, if your in-breath is 1 second, make your out-breath 2 seconds; if your inhale is 2 seconds, make your exhale 4 seconds. Breathe like this a few times to get the hang of it.**

4. **When you feel you've got it down, let your eyelids slowly close and continue with the doubled exhale for at least 10 breaths.**

5. **When you've reached 10 breaths, let your breathing return to normal and allow yourself to relax.**

This meditation encourages you to focus on your exhale so you can take advantage of its natural relaxing properties.

play with your breath

If you're feeling overly serious, frustrated, or down about your attempts to get some shut-eye, give this fun and playful meditation a try. Here's what to do:

1. Instead of following specific instructions (e.g., breathe in for this many seconds, breathe out this way), give yourself permission to play. The only rules are (1) to focus on your breath, and (2) to play with it.

2. You can lie down, sit up, stand up, or even bounce a little bit—whatever sounds like fun to you.

3. Pay attention to your breath and find a rhythm that feels fun and playful to you. Play with that rhythm for a while. You might take big, deep in-breaths and let out tiny exhales, or breathe in with short bursts and out with a wide-open mouth. Whatever you do, get a little silly and get a little loose.

4. As soon as it stops feeling fun, change it up. Continue until you feel it's been at least a few minutes or until you think you've blown off some steam.

5. Get into a comfortable sleeping position, take in 1 deep inhale, then let it out and relax into the bed.

Letting yourself get a little silly through this meditation might be just what you need to relax.

give gratitude for your breath

Gratitude has a host of benefits, including helping you get into a more relaxed, renewed state of mind. Adding a focus to your breath boosts this benefit, allowing you to shut down your busy brain and get back to sleep. Follow these instructions to build some gratitude for your breath:

1. Sit up with your eyes open and a soft focus. Take in a deep, long breath, breathing in for at least 4 seconds and out for at least 4 seconds.

2. Now, return to your normal breathing rhythm.

3. As you breathe in, think about how wonderful it feels to be able to breathe freely. If you've ever had a bad cold or lung infection, you know how it feels to struggle with obstructed breathing.

4. As you breathe out, focus on how easily you can exhale. Again, you'll know how great it feels to simply breathe out if you've ever had a bad cold with a stuffy nose.

5. Keep your mind on how grateful you are to be breathing freely as you inhale and exhale. Grow that sense of gratitude until you can't help but smile.

6. Take a few more deep breaths to close out the practice, then close your eyes and let yourself sink into sleep.

Gratitude is the foundation of peace, and peace is what will send you gently off to sleep.

breathe in a circle

This exercise is a good option if you are feeling overwhelmed and you have a little stiffness or soreness. It incorporates your breath with soft, gentle movement. Here's how it works:

1. Sit upright with your legs crossed and your back straight. Keep your eyes open at first.

2. Start moving your head slowly to one side, giving your neck a stretch. Go as far as feels comfortable for you.

3. Now, with your face looking either left or right, start moving your head up toward the ceiling. Then, you'll move your head toward your other side, and finally back down toward the floor, creating a big circle.

4. Try this movement with your eyes closed for maximum relaxation. If that makes you feel dizzy, no worries—just keep your eyes open.

5. Continue these big circles and match your movement to your breath, breathing in as you move from one side up and over to the other side, and breathing out as you move your head down and back to the beginning position. Move slowly so you don't rush your breath.

6. After 5 breaths, switch directions and continue moving and breathing steadily for another 5 breaths.

This is a great way to introduce some calm, whether you're trying to get to sleep or just feeling overwhelmed during your day.

visualize the breathing process

This meditation combines visualization with deep breathing to help you get relaxed and ready for sleep. Follow these steps to give it a try:

1. Lie down with your back flat on the bed and your legs out straight, arms by your sides.

2. Close your eyes and breathe in deeply, following your breath as it goes.

3. Visualize your breath moving in through your nose, down through your esophagus, and into your lungs. Watch as your lungs fill up like balloons.

4. As you exhale, watch your lungs deflate as the air rushes out, back up your esophagus and out through your nostrils.

5. See the process in detail, from the tiny hairs in your nose that flutter as the air passes, to the shiny, pink surface of the inside of your lungs as they inflate and deflate.

6. You might feel a sense of awe at your body working in such harmony to get the oxygen it needs. Let yourself feel that awe, and be grateful for the awesome way your body works.

7. Slow your breath and watch the process slow to match it. Allow it to soothe you into a relaxed, sleepy mindset.

This visualization is extra-helpful for the more "visual" people, but anyone can use it to introduce some sleepiness.

try "o" breathing

This silly-feeling exercise can help you relax and disengage your mind, getting you ready for sleep again. Follow these instructions to try "O" breathing:

1. In your comfortable meditation position, close your eyes and relax your body into whatever you are sitting or lying on.

2. Focus your attention on your breath, simply observing it as it goes in and out for a few moments.

3. Now, imagine you want to suck air through a large straw and change your mouth to a small "O" shape as you inhale. Inhale fully, filling your lungs.

4. As you exhale, relax your mouth into a natural shape.

5. Repeat this breath, making an "O" with your mouth as you breathe in and relaxing your mouth as you breathe out, for 5 breaths.

6. Next, switch to making an "O" shape when you breathe out and relaxing your mouth when you breathe in. Repeat for 5 breaths.

7. Notice how each technique makes you feel. If one is much more relaxing than the other, choose that technique and repeat for another 10 breaths.

Both techniques can help you focus on your breath and find peace, but breathing out with an "O" often helps release stress and induce calm as well.

breathe with your palm

This exercise combines a gentle hand movement with your breath to soothe and relax you. Turn on a soft light to get the full effect. Here's how it works:

1. In a comfortable seated position, look down at the palm of your nondominant hand (I'll use the left hand for this exercise). Place the pointer finger of your dominant hand at the base of your other hand, where your thumb meets your wrist.

2. Take a slow, deep breath in for 5 seconds as you move your finger up your palm toward the base of your pointer finger.

3. Hold your breath for 5 seconds as you drag your finger across your palm underneath your four fingers, ending up just below the pinkie finger on your left hand.

4. Exhale for 5 seconds as you drag your finger straight down to the heel of your hand.

5. Finally, hold for 5 seconds as you move your finger back to the starting position at the point where the base of your thumb and your wrist meet.

6. Repeat steps 2 through 5, breathing in, holding, breathing out, and holding as you move your finger around your palm.

Incorporating a visual element into this breathing exercise can be helpful for those who get distracted, and it connects your breath with slow, gentle movement.

use your core

You might automatically think of working out when you read "use your core," but you can also use your core to relax. This exercise engages your core to help you breathe more intentionally. Get comfortable, then follow these directions to give it a try:

1. Lie back on the bed and close your eyes. Take a few deep, relaxing breaths, in and out through your nose.

2. Place one hand on your belly. Take a few more breaths, breathing deeply in and out. Notice how it feels as your hand rises and falls with your breath.

3. Now, move your hand off your belly and place your other hand on your chest, just above your heart. Take a few more deep, soothing breaths. Pay attention to the rise and fall of your chest as you breathe.

4. Move your first hand back to your belly and keep your other hand on your chest. With both hands in place, breathe in and out, feeling the movement in your core as you do. Notice how it feels to breathe when you pay specific attention to your core.

5. See if you can slow your breathing any more. Take the longest, slowest breaths you've taken all day, feeling your chest and belly rise and fall as you do.

Focusing on your core can ground you in the present and prepare your mind for relaxation.

count your breaths—
forward and backward

Repetition can be soothing, and making "loops" can be even more so. Try combining the time-tested method of counting with intentional breathing and looping. Here's how it works:

1. Get into your favorite sleeping position in bed and settle in.

2. Turn your attention to your breath. Don't try to change it, just notice how it feels as you inhale and exhale. Do this for a few breaths.

3. Now, begin counting your breaths. Breathe in deeply, then count 1 on your exhale, whether in your head or out loud. Breathe in again, then count 2 on your next exhale. Keep counting until you get to 10.

4. Instead of continuing on to 11, go back down to 9. Continue counting backward until you get to 1.

5. Repeat these steps, looping your breath count up to 10, then back down to 1. Do at least 5 repetitions.

6. If you have repeated this loop 5 times and you're still feeling awake, increase your count to 20 breaths (i.e., counting up to 20 breaths and then back down to 1).

This exercise harnesses the power of looping along with counting the breath for an even more effective sleep aid.

breathe in color

Visualization is a powerful tool for inducing sleepiness, and adding it to this breath-based technique will help you get sleepier faster. Follow these instructions to give it a try:

1. **Get yourself into a comfortable position lying faceup on your bed, eyes open. You can have your knees up or down, your arms flung out wide or by your sides—whatever feels most comfortable and relaxing to you.**

2. **Bring your awareness to your breathing. Focus on the experience of breathing as you inhale and exhale.**

3. **Start to deepen and slow your breath. Inhale for a bit longer than you were originally and allow your exhale to stretch out a little longer.**

4. **Now, close your eyes and engage your imagination. On your next exhale, imagine you can see your breath. As it exits your nostrils, you see a puff of colorful air. You can choose whichever color feels relaxing and soothing to you, or you can simply see what color pops into your imagination. Watch as the colorful cloud swirls above your head and dissipates into the room.**

Colors have long been thought to have an effect on our mood or our energy state. Light pink, baby blue, and other pastel colors may be the most soothing, but it can depend on your preferences. You may even want to try a few different colors to see what is most relaxing for you.

use your breath to unload stress

Breathing exercises that focus specifically on your exhales can be very effective in releasing tension and inducing calm. Try using your breath specifically to unload your stress with this exercise:

1. Sit upright with your hands resting on your knees or thighs, palms facing up. Keep your eyes open to begin.

2. Take a few calming breaths as you settle into the bed.

3. When you feel ready, allow your eyes to gently close on an exhale.

4. With your eyes closed and your imagination on, see your body in your mind's eye. Notice the stress that's filling up your body. See it as a gently rippling liquid, and notice how far up it goes—perhaps up to your hips, your chest, or all the way to your head.

5. Now, with each breath you take, imagine you are unloading some of that stress. Watch as it exits your body through your nose and/or mouth. With each inhale, you are gathering up some of that stress. With each exhale, you are expelling that "liquid" from your body.

6. Continue breathing like this, inhaling to gather up stress and exhaling to unload it. Repeat until your body is completely free of stress.

This exercise is a great way to let go of stress and give your body and brain permission to relax.

try bee breathing

Bee breathing, also known as Bhramari Pranayama, is named for an Indian bee and uses breath, body sensation, and sound to invoke a sense of calm. Here's how it works:

1. Sit upright with your back straight and your eyes closed.

2. Place your thumbs on the cartilage between your ear and your cheek (i.e., as if you are going to close off your ears to sound). Place your index fingers above your eyebrows and your middle fingers on your eyelids. Rest your ring fingers gently on the sides of your nose and your pinkie fingers on your closed lips.

3. Breathe in steadily, feeling your nostrils flare as you inhale.

4. As you exhale, gently press your thumbs against the cartilage between your ears and your cheeks. Don't press too hard, just enough to muffle your hearing.

5. In addition to pressing on your cartilage with each exhale, introduce a humming sound as you breathe out (the "buzz" of your humming is where this technique gets its name).

6. Continue breathing in this manner for at least 10 breaths.

Notice how you feel after 10 breaths. If you're ready for sleep, keep your eyes closed as you slowly lie down and transition to sleep. If you're not tired yet, repeat this technique for another 10 breaths and reassess.

chapter two

body meditations

try progressive muscle relaxation

Sometimes, if you want to relax, it helps to tense up first. While this may seem counterintuitive, deliberately creating more muscle tension in your body will help you more fully and consciously release that tension. Follow these steps to give it a try:

1. Lie comfortably, flat on your back, with your arms by your sides.

2. Send all your energy down to your feet and use it to flex all your foot muscles. Scrunch your feet up as tightly as you can.

3. Hold this maximum tension for 3 seconds.

4. Let go of the tension, unflex your feet, and allow them to relax all the way.

5. Repeat this process with your calves, then your thighs, your hips and buttocks, your stomach and lower back, your chest and upper back, your fists and forearms, your upper arms, your shoulders and neck, and finally your face and head.

6. When you've finished flexing and releasing your entire body, feel how light and relaxed your body feels. Allow the relaxation to carry you back to sleep.

You may not realize how tight or anxious you are until you turn that body tension dial up to 11. Then you can intentionally turn the dial all the way back down to 0.

do a body scan

A body scan is a great way to get out of your head (and away from the thoughts running through it) and back into your body. You can also use what you learn from your body scan in another meditation focused on releasing tension or soothing a particularly tense part of your body. Here's how to do a basic body scan:

1. Make sure you're lying comfortably with your eyes closed. Breathe slowly and steadily in and out.

2. Send your awareness to the top of your head. Notice whether you are feeling any pain, tightness, itching, tingling, or any other sensation at the top of your head. Take note of what you feel.

3. Now, slowly drag your awareness down your body, noting how you feel as you go. Take your time with this, moving slowly and steadily from the top of your head all the way down to your toes.

4. Pay attention to the sensations you feel at each point in your body. Note the most salient or strongest sensations, like an especially tight or strained muscle.

Sometimes, just performing a quick body scan can help you be more present and relax into your body, preparing you for sleep. If you find any especially tight or tense parts, you can use another meditation to loosen them up and drift back to sleep.

power down your body

If you feel like your whole body is just too active and energized for sleep, doing a "power down" meditation can help you relax and let go of that nervous energy, getting you back into the right state of mind (and body) for sleep. Follow these instructions to give it a try:

1. Lie flat on your back in bed with your arms at your sides and your legs straight out. You can keep your eyes open at the beginning if you wish.

2. Starting with your feet and moving up to your head, "power down" your body, one portion at a time.

3. Feel your feet, humming with energy. Imagine an "on/off" switch that controls your feet, and flip it to "off." Feel the energy leave your feet and exit your body.

4. Continue up your legs, turning off your calves, your knees, your thighs, and so on, until you reach your head. Do not move any part of your body that you've already "powered down."

5. When you reach your head, power it down slowly by gently closing your eyes. When your eyes close, your head is completely powered down along with the rest of your body. Rest easy and allow yourself to drift back to sleep.

Like a robot who is instructed to "power down," you can use exercises like this to direct your brain to send relaxing signals to the rest of your body.

thank your body

A little gratitude can go a long way in a wide range of situations, including relaxing and settling in to sleep. Give your body some gratitude to help your busy brain shut off. Here's how:

1. Think about everything your body did for you today. List the many tasks your body carried out. Your list might include getting out of bed, showering, brushing your teeth, getting dressed, walking out to the car, driving to work, and walking into work—and that's all in the first few hours.

2. When you have a complete list in your mind, say "thank you" to your body for each task. For example, you might start with saying, "Thank you, body, for getting out of bed today." Continue thanking your body for each task it completed until you are through your entire list.

3. When you're out of tasks, give yourself a big mental hug and thank your body for carrying you through this day. Finally, give it permission to rest.

Your body does a lot for you. In fact, it "shoulders" the entire burden of carrying you through your day. Realizing how much stress you put your body through and giving it a little gratitude is a great way to de-stress and sink back into sleep.

give yourself a hug

You know how sometimes all you need to turn your day around is a hug from the right person? An embrace from a loved one can be just what we need to feel better. Consider that you are your own loved one, and the one who knows you best. Give yourself a hug to help you feel comforted, safe, and secure. Follow these instructions:

1. While sitting or lying comfortably, close your eyes and smile.

2. Lift your arms to shoulder height and slowly wrap them around your shoulders and upper arms.

3. Let them rest easily on your body for a few moments, then give yourself a little squeeze.

4. Repeat this process 5 times, letting your arms rest on your body followed by a comforting squeeze.

Humans are innately attuned to human touch. Giving yourself a warm, loving hug might be just what you need to create a sense of calm, comfort, and security that will gently rock you back to sleep. If you don't feel different after repeating this process 5 times, up it to 10 and see if anything changes. You might need a little extra self-love to get comfy enough for sleep.

give your body a break

Do you regularly give your body a purposeful break? We tend to get caught up in our minds instead of our bodies, but recognizing how tense our bodies can get may give us the key to stillness. To try giving your body a break, follow these steps:

1. **Lie down in whatever position is most comfortable for you, whether that's on your back, your side, or your stomach—just get cozy.**

2. **Wrap your arms around yourself, lock your hands together, put your hands to your cheeks, or do some other gesture that a loved one might do to comfort you.**

3. **Think about how it feels to be in your body right now. Notice any points of tension or stress.**

4. **Say to your body, "Body, thank you for carrying me through today. Now, take a break. Your job is done." Let all your muscles relax and allow your body to rest.**

Giving yourself a break is not only a good way to reduce tension; it also gives you permission to relax and be still. If you're still concerned about something you did, or you're thinking about a flaw, weakness, or mistake, try cultivating some self-compassion with the following two exercises.

send love to your favorite areas

If you have some insecurities or body image issues, you know that your body probably doesn't get as much love as it needs. To soothe your body, send some love to your favorite areas. Here's how:

1. With your eyes closed, picture your body in your mind's eye. See it in detail.

2. Choose three areas that you like, appreciate, or admire about your body. For example, you might choose your hair, your tummy, and your calves.

3. Gather up some love and good feeling for these three areas. Think about what you like about them and grow some nice, warm, fuzzy feelings.

4. One at a time, send these warm feelings to each area. Feel the warm, fuzzy love reach each area and infuse it with comfort and caring. Let it permeate the area and feel it in your very veins.

5. When you've sent love to all three areas, smile and give yourself a little hug (if that feels genuine to you).

Sometimes all we need to fully relax and drift off to a peaceful sleep is a little love and reassurance for our bodies. Beauty companies and gyms may try to convince you that there's something wrong with your body, but show yourself some love and you'll realize that it does exactly what you need it to.

send love to your flaws

If you've already tried the "Send Love to Your Favorite Areas" meditation, this one will feel familiar; it's similar, but this time you focus on your "flaws." In this context, a "flaw" can be anything that you don't really like about yourself, something that hasn't been cooperating, or something that's been causing pain—anything that isn't exactly a favorite body part at the moment. Here's how to send love to your flaws:

1. **Close your eyes and picture your body in your mind. Call up as much detail as you can.**

2. **Pick three areas that are bothering you. For example, if your ankle has been hurting lately, you might choose your ankle for one of the areas.**

3. **Put aside your frustrations and dislike of these three areas, just for a moment. In their place, conjure up some love. Think about how functional these areas have been (if not now, at least in the past), and how they've gotten you through to today.**

4. **Gather up some warm, fuzzy feelings and some gratitude, and send them to each area, one at a time.**

5. **Be open to the sensations as you send love. Feel the warmth and comfort as they travel through your body and soothe your area of choice. Repeat for each area.**

6. **Give yourself a smile and a little squeeze, then relax fully into the bed.**

Usually, when we think about our flaws, we get more anxious, upset, or frustrated; exercises like this one help you reframe and be more positive when you consider your "flaws."

play footsie with yourself

If you've ever played footsie with a crush or a loved one, you know it can be a silly, fun way to engage in playful physical touch. If you're trying to feel some peace and general good feeling in your body, playing footsie with yourself can be a helpful exercise. Here's how to do it:

1. Start lying down with your legs straight out. If it's chilly, you might want to put some socks on first. Make sure you're extra-cozy.

2. Slowly bring one foot up to rub against the other. Rub it down the top of the other foot a few times, all the way from ankle to toes. Next, rub it down the side a few times, then face the sole of the receiving foot toward the other so you can give the bottom of your foot a little rub.

3. Switch to the other foot, keeping that slow, gentle pace. Keep the mood light and silly, even imagining your feet as belonging to separate people who are actually flirting.

Sometimes it's easy to be playful and silly with others, but we may struggle to create that mood with ourselves. This exercise is a fun way to get out of your head and into your body, and show a little love for your body at the same time.

focus on what you feel

Most of us spend our days focused on what is going on in our heads, stuck in the past or present, and out of touch with our bodies. This meditation will help you focus on what you're feeling, as well as make you present and attuned to your body. Follow these instructions to focus on what your body is feeling:

1. **Whether you're sitting or lying down, let your muscles rest where they are. Don't try to sit up too straight or stretch out your legs—just relax.**

2. **With your eyes closed, try to clear away any strong or persistent thoughts. Let your mind be as blank and free as possible.**

3. **Bring your attention to your body. Cultivate awareness to catch any sensation your body is experiencing; that might be the feeling of your pajama pants against your leg, the feel of your sheet against your foot, or the sensation of the pillowcase against your cheek.**

4. **Send your full awareness to the sensations you feel. Notice each one and catalog it as if you were a scientist studying what it's like to feel things.**

5. **Close with a bit of gratitude for your ability to feel the world around you with your body.**

Getting out of your head and into your body is a nice way to prepare yourself for relaxation and let your mind rest.

give yourself a hand massage

A nice massage can take you from feeling tense and energetic to sleepy and content in less than an hour, but of course we don't all have access to a 24-hour masseuse. To give yourself a taste of the luxury and peace of a massage, try treating yourself to a hand massage. Here's how to do it:

1. Sit or lie in a position where you can easily move both hands.

2. Reach your dominant hand over to your other hand and clasp it gently. For the purposes of explaining this exercise, I'll start with the right hand as the massager and the left hand as the receiver.

3. Working slowly, start pressing your right thumb softly into the palm of your left hand. Move it in slow, gentle circles.

4. Now, move your thumb up through the center of your palm toward the webbing between your thumb and pointer finger. Knead upward, still moving slowly and gently.

5. Next, move your thumb down to the base of your left hand, just above the wrist. Rub slow circles into this part of your hand, moving from one side to the other.

6. Switch hands, making the left hand the massager and the right hand the receiver.

Letting yourself relax and feel a little pleasure is a great way to lull that stubborn mind back to sleep.

feel the warmth of the sun

This is an especially good exercise on a cold evening, but it can be used anytime. Humans are primed to welcome the sun as a source of life and support, making it a comforting and loving presence for most of us. Use this natural source of comfort to help you drift back to sleep:

1. **Cover yourself with a sheet or blanket if you're not already under the covers and get as warm as you can.**

2. **Close your eyes and think about the last time you felt the sun shining down on you. Call the memory to mind and be as detailed as possible. Note how it felt to soak in the warm, nourishing sunlight.**

3. **Imagine the sun shining down on you now, imparting all its warmth. Feel it as it seeps into you, through your skin, and into your very bones. Let it fill your body with a warm, loving, comforting feeling.**

4. **Imagine the sun melting away all your pain, your stress, and your troubles, and leaving you with just that sensation of warmth and comfort.**

As mentioned, this meditation is great for a cold day—even better if it's cold and rainy—but you can call on the warm, comfortable memory of the sun whenever you need a little extra coziness. Let it wash over you and lull you gently back to sleep.

get an imaginary massage

If you've ever had a gentle massage, you know it can get so relaxing that you have to fight to stay awake. It's not the same, but getting an imaginary massage can help you get back to sleep. Here's how:

1. **Lie flat on your stomach to start. Close your eyes and take in several deep, soothing breaths.**

2. **Imagine a massage therapist approaching you, folding the sheet down to access your back. Feel the sensations as the therapist begins to slowly massage your upper back, applying warm, aromatic oil as they go. Engage your sense of imaginary smell here as well as imaginary touch.**

3. **Bring in your sense of imaginary hearing as well, as you imagine soft, soothing music or nature sounds.**

4. **Feel the strong but gentle hands as they work up over your shoulders, down your back, and down your arms. Imagine the muscles releasing as the therapist massages down your legs and all the way to your feet.**

5. **Flip over onto your back and repeat the imagery with your front side. Feel the gentle massaging of your shoulders, biceps, forearms, and all the way down the top of your legs to your feet again.**

6. **Breathe deeply and sigh it out, relaxing into your bed.**

It may not be as effective as getting a real massage, but imagining one will send your body the message to relax and unwind.

put your cells to sleep

No matter how much they need their rest, children often fight falling asleep. Our bodies and minds can be the same way. Use this meditation to gently, lovingly put all your cells to sleep. Here's how to do it:

1. Sit or lie down with your eyes closed.

2. Engage your imagination. Visualize the cells in your body. It doesn't have to be an accurate representation. Maybe they look like tiny little versions of you, or maybe they look like amorphous blobs with your face on them. Whatever you're imagining, see it in detail.

3. Now, focus on the cells in one part of your body (for example, all the cells that make up your feet). Tell those cells that it's time for rest, and you're going to put them to sleep now. Imagine tucking them in with tiny blankets, and watch as they shut their eyes or slow their movement.

4. Repeat this visualization with another part of your body and continue until you have put the cells of all the different parts of your body to sleep.

5. Say a final goodnight and close your eyes as well, allowing your resting body to slip into a deep sleep.

Zooming in on your body can help you feel more gratitude for the amazing things it can do, putting you in a more positive and relaxed state of mind.

take a mental shower

Showers can be a great way to relax and prepare for sleep. But if you've already showered, you're out of hot water, or you can't indulge for another reason, you're not out of luck—you can take a mental shower to get your body ready for sleep. Here's how to take a mental shower:

1. **Lie down on your back with your eyes closed and your limbs stretched out long.**

2. **Imagine yourself getting up, walking over to the bathroom, and turning on your shower. Make it as hot as you like but still comfortable.**

3. **Watch yourself stepping into the shower and letting the water wash over your head and face. Engage your senses and feel the water as it hits your skin and slides all the way down your body to your feet.**

4. **Turn your face up to the showerhead and allow the water to gently fall on your face. Let it warm you up and make you feel clean all at once.**

5. **Imagine yourself standing under the running water for as long as you'd like. When you're ready, imagine yourself getting out of the shower, drying off, and walking back to bed. See yourself climbing into bed and, in sync with your visualized self, roll onto your favorite side and relax.**

Real showers can be super-relaxing, but you don't need to get wet to reap some of their soothing benefits.

give your face some love

The muscles in the face are often the most overworked and under-appreciated muscles. When you're stressed or overwhelmed, you probably carry tension in your face. Give your face a break and show it some love to soothe yourself back to sleep. Follow these steps:

1. If you haven't recently washed your hands, do so before you begin.

2. Reach your hands up to your face and let your palms rest gently on your cheeks, cupping your face.

3. Start moving your hands slowly in circles, pulling away from your face and toward your ears. Continue for a few breaths.

4. Now, place your hand on your forehead with your fingers pointing toward one another, just above your eyebrows. Gently pull back toward your ears, away from the center of your face, for at least a few breaths.

5. Finally, place the first three fingers of each hand on your temples and rub gently in slow, deliberate circles to relax your eyes.

6. Feel free to repeat any of these movements. When you're ready, try a gentle smile as you relax into sleep.

Even if you stay on top of exercising the muscles in the rest of your body (e.g., weight-lifting, Pilates) or soothing the muscles in the rest of your body (e.g., getting massages, yoga), most of us don't think about the muscles in our faces. Use this meditation to give them some love.

massage your scalp

Your head carries a lot of your stress, so try using your hands to relax your head and ease yourself back into sleep. Here's how:

1. Sit up in a comfortable position so you have access to your scalp.

2. Breathe in deeply and raise your hands up to your scalp as you exhale.

3. Take your hands and slide them up from the back of your head, just behind your ears, until they are cradling the back of your head.

4. Now, gently squeeze your hands inward, massaging the back of your head. Continue this motion for a few breaths.

5. Now, move your hands above your ears and upward, making your fingertips meet at the top of your head. Continue massaging this area for a few breaths.

6. Finally, place your hands on your head with the thumbs in front of your ears and your pinkies touching at the top of your forehead. Rub gently along your temples and all the way up your hairline.

7. Allow your hands to fall gently to your sides, lie down, and close your eyes to prepare for a relaxed sleep.

We store much of our tension in the head, so it makes sense to give it a little extra love if you want to float back to sleep.

stretch your sides

Use this stretching meditation to give your body some much-needed stretches and allow it to relax:

1. Lie flat on your back in your bed with enough space to stretch out a bit on either side.

2. Inhale deeply, filling your lungs entirely.

3. As you exhale, reach your arms above your head and stretch your whole body.

4. Take in another breath, then let it out as you reach your hands up and over to the left. Bring your feet over to the left as well, making your body into a banana shape.

5. Take 3 breaths here, feeling the stretch along the right side of your body.

6. Exhale and return to center.

7. Inhale again, then reach your hands and your feet over to the right as you exhale, making your body into a banana shape in the other direction.

8. Take 3 steady breaths as you hold this pose, stretching out the left side of your body.

9. Exhale and return to center.

10. Bring your arms down to your sides and allow your body to relax completely.

Even if you stretch often, you might forget the sides of your body. Try this exercise to give yourself a little extra stretch and relax your body enough for sleep.

be a starfish

This body-focused meditation is great for unwinding, especially if you're someone who usually gets "small" to sleep (e.g., curls up into a fetal position). Try this meditation to give yourself permission to be large, to take up space, and to own your space:

1. Lie down on your back with your eyes open and your arms and legs stretched out long.

2. Take a few calming breaths and allow your gaze to be soft and unfocused.

3. On an exhale, move your arms and legs into a wide star position. Stretch them out long, taking up space in your bed.

4. Hold the stretch for a few moments, breathing in and out deeply. Fill your lungs completely, then empty them completely.

5. Close your eyes and relax your body, but leave your arms and legs out wide. Feel how great it is to be large, to be present in this moment, and to be content.

6. Put a gentle smile on your face as you stretch your arms and legs out wide once more, reaching for even more space.

7. Finish by getting into your most comfortable sleeping position and relaxing completely.

Many of us tend to sleep in a tight little ball, but giving yourself permission to get out of your comfort zone is a great way to be kind and soothing to yourself.

rest in child's pose

If you're feeling anxious or troubled, this yoga pose is a great choice to soothe your busy mind and get you back into a sleepy state. Here's what to do:

1. Make some space on your bed to stretch out. If you don't have enough space, find a spot on the floor by your bed.

2. Sit upright, but with your knees out in front and your feet tucked under you.

3. Breathe in deeply, pause for a moment, then exhale completely. Repeat this deep breath 3 times.

4. On your last breath, lean forward as you exhale, all the way to the bed or floor. Stretch your arms out long over your head and let your body sink completely onto the tops of your thighs. If this feels a little uncomfortable, you can try moving your knees out wide instead.

5. Take a few relaxing breaths here, then move your arms down by your sides. Your shoulders should be by your knees and your hands down by your feet.

6. Take another big, deep breath in this pose. When you exhale, let go of all the stress, tension, and anxiety.

7. Stay here as long as you'd like, then make your way to your favorite sleeping position.

This classic yoga pose will help you find peace and relaxation.

drink an imaginary sleeping potion

If you're having trouble getting to sleep, try imagining that you've taken a sleeping potion and manifesting the effects. Here's what to do:

1. Lie back but keep your eyes open for now. Engage your imagination.

2. Think about how it would feel in your body to take a sleeping potion. Would it move through your bloodstream slowly or quickly? How would it make your muscles feel? How would it influence your thinking patterns?

3. Pretend that you just took a sleeping potion. However you think a sleeping potion would work, imagine that you are feeling the effects now.

4. Follow it as it moves through your body, quieting any nervous energy and soothing your muscles into relaxation. Feel it as it permeates your torso, flows down your legs and up your arms. Imagine a slight tingling in your veins as it works its way through your body.

5. Feel its effects as your eyes gently shut, too heavy to stay open. Slow your breathing and relax completely.

Sometimes pretending or imagining yourself to be sleepy can convince your busy brain that you really are sleepy, and get you back to your slumber.

try a few yawns

Yawning is the universal sign of being tired, and your brain knows that. If you're not sleepy but you want to be, forcing a few yawns can give your brain the "I'm sleepy" message it needs to get you back to a sleepy state of mind. Here's how to do it:

1. Get comfy on your bed but start in a seated posture.

2. Close your eyes and breathe steadily, preparing your lungs for some big breaths.

3. Take a deep breath in, hold it for a moment, then exhale it out completely.

4. As you go to inhale, force yourself to yawn instead. As you yawn, breathe in deeply, completely filling your lungs. Open your mouth as wide as possible at the top of the yawn.

5. Send all that air whooshing out as you exhale out your mouth, then close it. Take another deep breath, no yawn this time.

6. Repeat these steps, taking a preparatory deep breath, then switching to a big yawn, then taking another recovery breath. Follow this pattern 5 times, for a total of five yawns.

7. On your final yawn, let yourself fall back into your bed as you exhale, then take your final recovery breath in your favorite sleeping position.

Did you know that yawns really are contagious? Use this exercise to be the source and the mimicker.

rub your tummy

It sounds funny, but rubbing your stomach can be a very soothing and relaxing exercise for your body and brain. Follow the instructions to put yourself to sleep using your tummy:

1. Lie back with your hands at your sides and your eyes open.

2. Take a deep breath in through your nose and out through your mouth. Make it a big breath, filling up your lungs completely and exhaling with gusto.

3. Now, place your hands on your stomach and close your eyes. Feel your belly rise and fall as you breathe in and out.

4. Start slowly rubbing your belly, moving in a circular motion with both hands.

5. After a few moments, start to apply a bit of pressure. Don't push hard enough to cause discomfort, but think about trying to massage the muscles and organs underneath the skin.

6. Experiment with hand movements and find a way to rub your stomach that feels good for you. Continue rubbing as you breathe in deeply, in through your nose and out through your nose, for 10 breaths.

The muscles in your stomach rarely get the luxury treatment that your back and shoulders do during massages. Give them some love, and you'll soothe your body to a sleepy state of mind.

try soothing, repetitive motion

This exercise combines mindfulness and repetitive motion—two ingredients sure to produce a mind that's ready for sleep. Here's how to give it a try:

1. **Think of a motion that you can do repeatedly for at least a few minutes without getting tired or frustrated. You might choose slowly stroking your arm with your hand, gently rocking back and forth, or anything else that feels easy and soothing to you.**

2. **Get into a cross-legged position on your bed and close your eyes. Whatever movement you chose, start doing it. For this example, I'll use rocking back and forth.**

3. **Gently lean forward as far as is comfortable for you, then slowly lean back about as far. Continue rocking slowly forward and backward.**

4. **Find a rhythm that feels comfortable, then match your breath to it. For example, you may want to breathe in for 2 "rocks" and breathe out for 2 "rocks."**

5. **Continue rocking to this rhythm for 10 breaths or until you feel your mind starting to relax.**

Repetitive motion has long been a method for soothing. Its roots go all the way back to being rocked by your caregivers when you were an infant. You might not have anyone to rock you to sleep now, but you can give yourself the same feelings by mimicking the same movement.

get into reclined cobbler's pose

If you've never heard of this pose, don't worry; it's a simple one. This exercise will walk you through how to use it to induce a sense of calmness:

1. First, make sure you have some room on your bed. If you have a very small bed or you are sharing the bed, find some space on the floor.

2. Lie down with your knees bent and the soles of your feet on the bed or ground.

3. Slowly let your knees fall out to the sides, joining the soles of your feet together. This will make a diamond shape out of your legs. (Don't worry, it's okay if you can't get your legs down to the bed or ground; if it's uncomfortable, bolster your outer thighs with two pillows.)

4. Once you're comfortable, turn your attention to your breath. As you breathe in, gather calm, soothing energy. As you breathe out, direct this energy toward your inner thighs, allowing the muscles to get even deeper into the stretch.

5. Place your hands either on your thighs, encouraging them to relax even more toward the bed or ground, or place them on your belly so you can feel it rise and fall with your breath. Continue in this pose for 10 breaths, then roll into your favorite sleeping position.

If you feel like it, you can add a final touch: Say "thank you" to your feet for carrying you all day, and allow them to rest.

use lion's breath

If you like feeling silly and have some tension to release, this is a great option. Here's how to do it:

1. Get into a comfortable seated position with your legs crossed and your hands resting on your knees. Keep your eyes open.

2. Breathe in deeply through your nose and exhale through your mouth. Repeat this breathing method for 5 breaths.

3. Next, breathe in deeply just like you've been doing; however, on your exhale, open your mouth, stick out your tongue, and turn your gaze up toward the center of your forehead (also known as your third eye). It will probably feel really silly and maybe even difficult at first, but stick with it.

4. Repeat this technique for 10 breaths, exhaling forcefully each time.

5. After your tenth lion's breath, return to breathing deeply in through the nose and out through the mouth. Continue like this for 5 breaths.

6. Lie back, close your eyes, and begin inhaling and exhaling through your nose. Allow your breath to return to its natural rhythm and drift off to sleep.

As odd as it sounds—and looks—this technique lets you get rid of stress and unload any extra energy, making it easier to enter a sleepy state of mind.

press out stress

When you feel too stressed or agitated for sleep, focusing on soothing your body is a great way to soothe your mind as well. Here's how to do it:

1. Sit up with your back resting against the wall, the headboard, or a pillow. You should be able to reach your thighs and shins with your hands (it's fine to bend your legs if you need to).

2. Breathe in deeply through your nose and exhale slowly through your mouth. Repeat a few times.

3. Now, move your hands to your thighs. Apply gentle pressure as you glide your hands toward your knees. Close your eyes and imagine you are pressing the tension and stress from your thighs down.

4. Repeat this soothing, gentle motion for a few moments, allowing your thigh muscles to relax, then move your hands to your shins and repeat the motion. Imagine the stress being pushed down toward your feet.

5. Continue pressing out the stress for a few more moments, then move on to your feet and complete the action. See all of your stress leaving your body through your feet as you give yourself a soothing foot rub.

This exercise will help you actually *feel* the stress leave your body, leaving nothing but peace behind.

pile on the pillows

If you have ever relaxed under a weighted blanket, you know how soothing it can be to have some extra weight on you. This exercise uses props to mimic that comforted feeling. Here's how to do it:

1. Before getting into a comfortable position on your bed, gather up a few pillows and place them beside you. If you have a body pillow, make sure that is within arm's reach as well. If you don't have many pillows, grab a blanket or two or even some towels—anything that you can use to add weight.

2. Lie back and get comfy, pulling your covers over you.

3. Close your eyes and begin to deepen your breath.

4. After a few relaxing breaths, reach over to your pile of pillows and blankets and grab one, moving it on top of you. Take another slow breath in and out, feeling the difference in your breath with the added weight.

5. Reach out and grab another pillow or blanket, and gently place that on top of the first one. Again, take a deep breath, focusing on how different it feels to inhale and exhale with the extra weight on top of you.

6. Continue adding pillows or blankets until you feel the maximum coziness.

Once you are comfortable, take a few minutes to simply breathe, focusing on how it feels to breathe under the weight of the pillows.

reverse the blood flow

If you've never tried meditating in a position other than sitting or lying down, this can be a fun way to try something new, while also relaxing and preparing your body for rest. Read on to give it a try:

1. Sit on the edge of your bed with your feet flat on the floor and your hands resting on your thighs or your knees.

2. Breathe in deeply through your nose and out through your mouth. Repeat this breath 3 times.

3. Close your eyes and lean forward, reaching toward putting your head between your knees. It's okay if you don't make it all the way; the goal is to get your head below your heart.

4. With your head between your knees, feel the sensations of your blood pumping through your head. Your face and neck might feel a little warmer, even flushed. You might even feel your heartbeat throb in your head.

5. Take 10 slow, steady breaths in this position. Note how it feels to breathe in and out in such a different position.

6. After 10 breaths, slowly bring your head up until you're sitting upright again. You might feel a slight head rush as you do. If you do, stay present and note the sensations.

7. Take a few more calm, relaxing breaths, then lie back and get ready for sleep.

Make sure not to push too far if you get uncomfortable. Stop whenever it feels right to you.

kick your feet up

If you need a little help relaxing, kick your feet up—literally. Putting your feet above your heart is a great way to encourage a soothing, relaxing energy flow in your body. Follow these steps to give it a try:

1. **Grab an extra pillow or two—ones you won't be using for your head—and have them nearby, then lie back with your head on your usual pillow.**

2. **Close your eyes and breathe slowly and steadily, in through your nose and out through your mouth. Repeat for 5 breaths.**

3. **Now, reach over and grab your extra pillow or two. Place them underneath your feet and calves, so your lower legs feel propped up and supported.**

4. **Lean back with your head resting comfortably on your pillow. If you opened your eyes, close them again.**

5. **Take several minutes to simply breathe and notice how this pose feels. As you breathe steadily in and out, note how it feels to have your feet up and to feel extra support underneath your legs. Pay attention to your heartbeat and notice if it slows at all with your feet up.**

6. **Remove the extra pillows and prepare for sleep.**

After you finish this meditation, take note of your thoughts and your mood; notice if you feel more mentally or emotionally supported, just as your legs were physically supported.

chapter three
thought meditations

let your mind be the sky

You might have trouble falling asleep because you get caught up in your thoughts. They come in and out of your head at will, sometimes at lightning speed, and it feels like there's nothing you can do but helplessly follow them as they come.

You can't help what thoughts come up, but you do have a choice about what to do with them. This exercise encourages you to let your thoughts come and go like clouds. Think about how you watch clouds: You don't obsessively follow one cloud; you simply watch it until it fades from view and move your gaze to a new cloud. In this exercise, that's exactly what you do; your thoughts become like clouds in the sky of your mind, floating past without bothering or troubling you. If you're struggling with wayward and unmanageable thoughts, follow these steps:

1. **Let your mind be blank and allow any thought that pops into your head to be there.**

2. **Now, try "thought-watching": Watch one thought as it enters your mind and passes by, like a cloud.**

3. **Don't chase away or shame the thought, but don't latch on to it either. Simply note it and let it float past.**

4. **Wait for another thought to float past and continue thought-watching.**

This exercise can be challenging at times, but that's when it's best to practice. You'll be a pro at thought-cloud-watching in no time!

think big, feel small

If you're feeling overwhelmed or bogged down by what's happening in your life at this moment, it can help to broaden your perspective. Try thinking big to feel small, allowing yourself to take the pressure off and drift into a peaceful sleep:

1. Take a few deep breaths to center yourself. Clear your mind as best you can.

2. Find the edges of your current awareness. (Hint: Your awareness is probably on just your mind and body right now.)

3. Expand that awareness out to the room around you. Think about what is happening in the room (e.g., a fan is blowing air, a pet is napping).

4. Expand your awareness to the house, apartment, or building you are in. Think about what is happening in this space (e.g., a family member is cooking, a coworker is on a phone call).

5. Expand even farther to the town or city you are in, and think of all the things happening there.

6. Continue expanding farther and farther, until you get all the way to the earth itself, then the galaxy, then the universe. Think about all that is happening in the universe, and how small your part is. Prepare yourself for sleep.

This meditation will help you let go of the hold you have on your anxieties or troubles, and revel in feeling small.

try loving-kindness meditation

This type of meditation is beloved by people all around the world for its ability to create calm, contentedness, and care. These are the steps:

1. Sit comfortably with your hands resting gently on your knees and your eyes open.

2. Take in a few slow, steady breaths, in through the nose and out through the mouth.

3. Close your eyes as you exhale, then switch to breathing in and out through the nose.

4. Find a spark of love and kindness within you. Feed it as you would a fire, allowing it to grow. Feel the love and kindness you have for yourself and allow it to suffuse you.

5. Now, add more to the loving-kindness fire and expand it outward to the people you love. Share the good feelings.

6. Put even more love and care into it and expand it to cover all the people you know—even those you don't like. Let it reach to each of them, carrying love with it.

7. Finally, expand it to all living beings on earth. Say to yourself, "May all living things be happy and free of suffering."

8. Sit with this loving feeling for a few moments longer, then lie down and snuggle into your bed.

Loving-kindness is a reminder to be positive when the world is getting you down.

meditate on your past

Meditation is about being present, but you can still be present in your mind while stepping away from current stressors. Let go of your present frustration by following these steps:

1. Put aside any frustration or irritation for the moment. You can always come back to it later if you choose to.

2. Think about the events in your life that brought you to this current moment. What are the biggest milestones in your life thus far?

3. Focus on the opportunities you've had for growth and the things that have built your character. Give a silent "thank you" for these events that have made you stronger.

4. Now, think about the things that you have enjoyed most— your favorite days and the moments that made them great. Give another silent "thank you" for each of these moments.

5. See that your life is full of ups and downs, as all lives are. Know that without these events in your past, you would not be who you are today or where you are today.

6. Acknowledge that everything in your life has led you to this moment, so it must be the "right" moment for you. Accept this truth and allow your frustrations over the past to slip away. Give yourself permission to simply be, and relax into the present moment.

Letting go of the past isn't always easy, but it's always worth it.

meditate on your present

Sometimes the present can feel overwhelming or frustrating. This is especially true when your mind or body refuses to cooperate, like when you want to go back to sleep. Try approaching your present in a different way to allow your brain to relax enough for slumber. Here's how:

1. Sit upright with your back straight and your hands resting on your knees. Keep your eyes open.

2. Take a few deep, relaxing breaths.

3. Think about how you got to your present moment, and spend a minute or two in gratitude for your past that brought you here (the exercise "Meditate On Your Past" in this chapter can help you with this part).

4. Now, come back to the present. Breathe in. Look around you, noting the things that are part of the present moment. Ground yourself in the present, and draw in inspiration from what is around you.

5. Take another minute or two for gratitude, but focus it on the present moment instead of the past. Give thanks for being where you are today.

6. Finally, surrender to the present moment and lie back, getting comfy in your bed.

We often struggle to be in the present moment, especially when feeling frustrated. Use this meditation to find peace in the present.

meditate on your future

If you find it difficult to appreciate the present moment for some reason, it might help to look ahead instead. Focusing on what's coming up for you instead of what's bothering you right now can ease the pressure and allow your mind to rest. Here's how to look ahead:

1. **Lie comfortably but keep your eyes open with a soft gaze.**

2. **Ask yourself the classic interview question: "Where do you see yourself in five years?"**

3. **Without the pressure of answering this question to an interviewer's satisfaction, relax and think about it. Where do you think you'll be? Who do you think will be in your life? What will you be doing?**

4. **When you have an image of where you will be in five years, think about the steps you will take to get there. Perhaps you will move to a new city, get a new job, or meet someone important.**

5. **As you think about the good things in your future, rest easy. Know that all of these blessings are on their way, and that it's meant to be. Release the pressure from yourself to do anything in particular *right now*.**

6. **Get into your favorite sleeping position and allow yourself to let go and fully relax into the bed.**

Thinking ahead to a positive place will get your brain into a positive state of mind now, allowing you to slip into sleep.

do a thought experiment

If your brain simply isn't ready for sleep yet, it might want to do some work first. Give it a job to do by running a thought experiment. Here's how to do it:

1. In a comfortable position—either seated or lying down—keep your eyes open and look upward (it helps you think creatively).

2. Pick a dilemma or problem you're currently facing. For example, you might think about how you've felt more bored than usual lately.

3. Think of at least three different ways you could solve this problem. For example, if you're feeling bored, you might consider trying kickboxing, networking to find better work opportunities, or starting a gratitude practice.

4. For each scenario, run through what would happen if that's how you moved forward. How would your life change? How would you change? What would you like about your new life? What new challenges would you face?

5. Think about whether you want to move forward with any of your ideas. If so, rest easy. If not, that's okay—know that you did some good thinking anyway.

Thought experiments are not only fun and interesting; they can also distract you from frustration—like when you are fretting over your sleeplessness.

learn to surrender

Many of us have trouble letting go. We cling tightly to the idea that we are in charge of what happens in our life and we can direct our own path. You do have choices, of course, but you also need to acknowledge that you can't control everything. Use this meditation to practice surrendering—allowing yourself to let go and drift off to sleep:

1. **Start sitting up, with a straight back and your hands resting on your knees. Your eyes can be open or closed.**

2. **Think about the present moment. Consider how you got here; surely your path is peppered with conscious decisions you made, but note the coincidences, the accidents, and the "acts of fate" that also brought you here.**

3. **Consider that if one small event had happened differently— if you didn't bump into the person who eventually became your partner, if you didn't take that job that you were undecided on at first, or if you were raised in a house one block down the street—you would probably be in a completely different place.**

4. **Realize that we have little control over what happens to us, only how we respond to what happens to us.**

5. **Choose to give up the need to feel in control and instead surrender to the moment.**

Let go, and you will feel your burden immediately lightened.

put your thoughts to bed

When your mind is busy with thoughts in the middle of the night, it can be tough to quiet them down and get back to sleep. Try this meditation to lovingly put those thoughts to rest. Here's how:

1. Get comfortable and begin by taking the deepest breath you've taken all day. Fill your lungs completely, then exhale and empty your lungs completely. Repeat this deep breath 3 more times.

2. Now, identify the thoughts that are bouncing around in your head, making it hard to shut off your brain.

3. Imagine taking one of these thoughts and lovingly tucking it into bed. See yourself taking hold of the thought, giving it a little hug, and putting it into bed. Pull the covers up over it and tell it "Goodnight."

4. Repeat this process for each of the stray thoughts you have, treating them gently and tucking them in as you would a beloved child.

5. When all of your thoughts have been tucked into bed, tuck yourself into bed as well with a clear head and a relaxed mind.

It can be easy to get frustrated when your mind is busy with thoughts, but treating your thoughts gently and lovingly will help you take the pressure off and relax your mind back into a sleepy state.

think about your sleeping success

If you're struggling to fall asleep, it can be helpful to think back to all the many, many times you've successfully fallen asleep in the past. You've done it before, and you can do it again. Here are the steps:

1. Adopt a seated posture to lessen the pressure you may be feeling to get back to sleep.

2. Think back to a time when you were very, very tired. Remember how easily you succumbed to sleep.

3. Now, think about all the times you went to bed and fell fast asleep without even thinking about it. It wasn't hard or easy; it was just something that you did.

4. Now, think about a time when you struggled to get to sleep, when you just couldn't sleep no matter what you did. Remember that, eventually, you did fall asleep.

5. Consider the wide range of experiences we all have with sleep, from "can't keep your eyes open" to "can't sleep no matter what." Sleep might not be easy right now, but you can be sure that it will be again at some point.

6. End the meditation with a deep breath and a smile.

Be thankful for the times when sleep came easy to you, and remind yourself that this difficulty getting back to sleep is temporary.

imagine life without sleep

When you're having trouble getting to sleep, you might focus too intently on the idea of sleeping. Loosening your focus on sleeping can get your mind off of your inability to sleep and on to relaxation. Here's how to loosen your focus on sleeping:

1. Lie flat on your back with your eyes open and a soft gaze up toward the ceiling.

2. Ask yourself this question: "What would life be like without sleep?"

3. Let your imagination run wild answering this question. Think about how you would spend the extra 8-ish hours a day. Ask yourself silly questions like "Would everyone still have a bed?" or "Would alarm clocks ever have been invented?" Consider this fictional world in detail.

4. Continue imagining what it would be like never to need sleep again, to have zero pressure to get to sleep. Let this imagined state of mind sink in, and pretend that *you* don't need to sleep either.

5. Tell yourself you can choose whether you want to sleep or not. If you're ready, get comfy and choose to get back to sleep. If you're not, get up to do a quiet, relaxing activity (like reading or stretching).

Engaging your imagination is great for the mind, and it can lull you back to a sleepy state.

simply be present

The ability to be present in the moment is an incredibly valuable skill to have. Being present is about rooting your mind in the current moment—not the past, not the future, but right here and right now. Aside from all the other benefits, learning to be present can also help you relax into sleep. Practice being present to get back to sleep with these steps:

1. Adopt whatever posture is comfortable and feels natural to you, but keep your eyes open.

2. Think about where you are and what you are doing in this moment. Say it to yourself. For example, you might say, "It's late at night and I'm sitting on my bed."

3. Breathe in and out steadily as you look at your surroundings.

4. Pay attention to your thoughts. They will probably quickly turn to the past or present; for example, they might go to "I need to fall asleep or I'll be tired tomorrow" or "I wish I had done better on X task earlier today." When they do, turn them gently back to the present moment by repeating the preceding acknowledgment.

5. Continue staying present for a few minutes, then breathe out, close your eyes, and let your mind drift off.

Practice being present often, and you will reap the benefits, one of which is finding it easier to relax and fall asleep.

use a sound machine

Many people use a sound machine to help them get to sleep. The white noise might keep your mind from getting too busy and help you feel relaxed. Follow these steps to use a sound machine to get back to sleep:

1. Turn on your sound machine and choose a sound that's relaxing to you. If you don't have a sound machine, use an app or browser to pull up a soothing soundtrack on your phone.

2. Sit comfortably with your blanket or comforter pulled up around you and close your eyes.

3. Breathe in deeply, and as you exhale, focus your attention on the sound you chose to play.

4. Notice each of the distinct sounds you can hear. For example, if you chose a rainforest sound, notice the birds cawing, frogs croaking, rain gently falling, etc.

5. Create an image of the place where you might hear these sounds. Think about the positive feelings this place engenders in you, like contentment, curiosity, or joy.

6. Bring yourself back to the present moment, but take those feelings with you. Continue listening to the sounds for a few moments, then open your eyes and lie down.

You can use all of your senses to help you relax and rejuvenate, so don't forget to give your ears some love.

normalize your experience

Tough times can be doubly tough when you feel bad about feeling bad. Instead of chastising or getting down on yourself, try normalizing what you're feeling to promote a sense of peace and get back to a sleepy state of mind. Here's how:

1. Take a few deep, cleansing breaths to clear your head.

2. Think about what you are feeling right now. Identify each of the feelings and label them so you know what you're dealing with.

3. Think about what you're up against or the things you're struggling with. Make a mental list if that helps.

4. Remind yourself that anxiety, unease, anger, or whatever else you're feeling right now are totally normal ways for a person to feel in the face of these challenges.

5. Tell yourself that you're normal, and that you're okay. It's perfectly fine to feel the way you feel right now. But know that this will eventually pass.

6. Now that you know your feelings are normal, take a big, deep breath and exhale loudly, letting it all go.

When you're distressed or frustrated, you might unintentionally make things worse by telling yourself you're alone in these feelings or there's something wrong with you. Ditch those negative thoughts, and you'll find yourself calmer and sleepier.

create a thought safe space

Safe spaces can be helpful for a variety of purposes, including promoting peace and calm. Try creating a safe space for your thoughts to quiet your mind and soothe yourself back to sleep. Follow these steps:

1. **Get cozy and comfortable, then close your eyes and take 1 deep breath. Try to clear your mind of extra thoughts, but don't worry if that's hard right now—we'll work on clearing out some of those thoughts.**

2. **Build a new space in your mind. As you build this space, keep the specifications in mind; it has to (1) hold your thoughts safely and securely, and (2) be a judgment-free zone. There is no judgment, shaming, or chastising of thoughts allowed here. Your thoughts are free to exist however they are in this space.**

3. **Once you have your safe space, take all the thoughts you have that you'd rather not have and put them here. If you have a thought that makes you feel ashamed, confused, or surprised at yourself, put it here.**

4. **With those thoughts safely tucked away in their safe space, breathe a sigh of relief and allow yourself to relax. Your thoughts are secure and cannot harm anyone, not even you.**

Feel free to return to the safe space to consider these difficult thoughts when you're in the right frame of mind to do so.

imagine the vastness of space

Thinking about the sheer size and complexity of our universe is a great way to get some perspective...and perspective might be just what you need to get out of your busy mind and into a sleepy state. Here's how to take advantage of this celestial sleep aid:

1. Lie back in a comfortable position and close your eyes.

2. Bring your awareness to the space above you. Picture what the night sky looks like overhead. See the shining stars, comets, and planets twinkling on the dark backdrop of space.

3. Now, take your awareness up into space and explore a little. Take a mental tour of the Milky Way galaxy (our home galaxy).

4. After a minute or two of exploring, once you've gotten a feel for how vast the galaxy is, remind yourself of this fact: The Milky Way is one of about two *trillion* galaxies in the known universe.

5. Think about what a teeny, tiny little drop in the bucket our galaxy is in the vastness of space, let alone our planet or the room we're currently in.

6. With stars in your (closed) eyes, appreciate the broader perspective while you allow your body to relax fully into your bed, ready for sleep.

Feeling small and insignificant may not sound like a good thing, but it certainly can be with this exercise.

set an intention

If you've taken yoga classes or meditated before, this process might be familiar to you. Setting an intention is a great way to direct your thoughts where you'd like them to go and manifest what you want. Try setting an intention when you want to get back to sleep. Here's how:

1. **Start by sitting upright with your hands on your knees. You can leave your eyes open with a soft focus or let them close.**

2. **Ask yourself what you want to do. Of course, the answer is probably "I want to fall back to sleep." But what needs to happen for you to fall asleep? Two things: (1) Your body needs to relax, with your muscles at ease. (2) Your mind needs to power down.**

3. **Now that you know what needs to happen, set an intention that will bring about these two preconditions for sleep. It might be something like "Create a sense of peace" or "Set aside the worries and anxieties currently on my mind." Or, it might be just one word, like "serenity."**

4. **With your intention in mind, close your eyes and focus on your breath. Will your intention into being with your breath, and return to it whenever you get distracted.**

5. **Continue for 10 breaths or until you feel ready for sleep.**

Setting an intention can help you get back to sleep and can also help with just about any goal you have.

note your thoughts

This simple technique of observing your thoughts is good for a lot of things—including getting your mind ready for slumber. Here's how:

1. Get comfortable and settle in with some steady breathing.

2. Once you're settled, bring your awareness to whatever thoughts are bouncing around your head right now.

3. When you observe each thought, simply note that it is a thought that you are currently having. Act like a curious researcher, taking notes. You don't feel connected to the thought; you are simply seeing it and noting that fact.

4. Once you note the existence of a thought, move on to another one. Don't spend too long noting any particular thought. Take note and continue scanning.

5. Continue noting your thoughts for a few minutes.

6. After those few minutes are up, turn your attention back to your breath. Observe how it feels to breathe deeply, in and out, for 3 breaths.

7. Finally, open your eyes and move into a comfortable sleeping posture, ready for sleep to overtake you.

It might seem too simple to work, but just noticing your thoughts can be incredibly soothing for a mind that tends to quickly jump from one thought to the next.

practice visual mindfulness

If you're the type of person who struggles to sit still with eyes closed, this meditation can help you settle and soothe your mind. Follow these instructions to try visual mindfulness:

1. Get into a comfy posture and leave your eyes open.

2. Take a deep, full breath in and exhale completely. Let your breath return to a normal, steady rhythm.

3. Now, look slowly around the room you're sitting in. What do you see? Your mind will probably notice the big things first: a bed, a chair, a dresser, a mirror, etc. Take note of all of these things as your gaze wanders over them.

4. Now, take another sweep through the room, this time looking for the smaller things: a small chip out of the paint in your wall, a book on the shelf, a quarter on your nightstand, etc. See all the things you don't normally see.

5. Now, do another sweep of the room, this time focusing on colors. Take note of all the different colors in the room.

6. Look around your room once again, now noticing all the different shapes of objects in the room.

7. Continue focusing on different aspects of things in your room, whether it's texture, type of object, size, etc.

This simple exercise in observing and noting what is around you will tune you in to the present moment and give your mind something to do instead of sitting and idly waiting for sleep.

ask yourself what you want

If you can't get back to sleep, try asking yourself an important question and pondering the answer to give your brain something to do—other than worrying about getting to sleep. Here's what to do:

1. Start with a quick breathing exercise to get in the right mindset. Breathe in for 3 seconds, pause for a moment, and breathe out for another 3 seconds. Take another brief pause, then repeat for 5 breaths.

2. With a cleared mind, ask yourself this question: "What do you want?" Ask it as it's worded, not from a first-person perspective (e.g., not "What do *I* want?"), and don't expand on or add anything to the question (e.g., not "What do you want *from life*?").

3. Notice where your mind goes. Don't worry about what actually comes up; instead, focus on how your mind goes about answering the question. Does it go to the broader perspective ("from life") or the narrower perspective ("in this moment")? Does it ponder material things (like "a house") or intangible things (like "freedom")?

4. Follow your mind for a while, noting the paths it takes. If you get distracted, bring your focus back to the question.

5. Repeat the breathing exercise from step 1, then end the meditation.

The simple act of asking and answering yourself can be an excellent tool to getting your mind to do what you suggest and get back to sleep.

be curious

Being curious is a great way to step back from any distress or tension and get into a calm, nonjudgmental state of mind. Follow these steps to use your curiosity to soothe your mind:

1. Get into a comfortable seated position but leave your eyes open. Take a calming breath, breathing in for 4 seconds, pausing, then breathing out for 4 seconds.

2. Turn your attention to what you're thinking about right now. Is your mind jumping from one thought to the next? Or is it holding on to one thought?

3. Now, turn your attention to what you're feeling. Are you feeling more agitated or relaxed? Are you feeling multiple things at once? What are you feeling?

4. What do you think is causing you to feel this way? Are you simply reacting to waking up in the middle of the night, or is there something else influencing you?

5. Use these questions—and more questions, if they come up—to explore your current experience. Think about how your mind is working right now and what that says about your mind in general. Stay curious and open-minded.

6. End the session with another 4-second breath and close your eyes, ready for sleep.

Curiosity may have been fatal for the feline, but it can be used to calm your busy human mind.

count your thoughts

If your mind is moving a mile a minute, don't fret—there are things you can do to soothe your busy mind and relax into sleep. Counting sheep might be challenging, but you can try counting your thoughts. Here's how to try this meditative exercise:

1. Adopt whatever posture is most comfortable right now. Set a timer with a quiet notification sound for 5 minutes, and close your eyes.

2. Picture your mind as a big, dark, empty space. Imagine that when you have a thought, it zips through this space with a flash of light. This allows you to see all the thoughts that come up against the dark backdrop of your mind.

3. Next, pick a spot in your mind and settle in to watch the thoughts. Notice when they come up, and don't engage or follow them; simply count each one as it flashes in the dark.

4. Continue counting thoughts until your timer goes off. If you get distracted, simply start again at 1. When the notification sounds, turn the timer off and close your eyes again.

5. Now, bring your attention to your breath. Take a few deep, slow, soothing breaths.

This meditation is a great way to detach from your thoughts. It also gives your busy brain something to do instead of fixating, which helps it relax.

follow a belief

When you're wide awake at a time you'd rather be asleep, one of the best things you can do to distract yourself and relax is to do some critical thinking. Try this meditation to do some critical thinking about your own beliefs:

1. Get in a comfortable meditation position, close your eyes, and open your hands, palms up.

2. Think about what beliefs you hold that may not be accurate and choose one to explore. The deeper and more closely held, the better. For instance, you may choose a belief like "I must be successful to be happy."

3. Now, follow this belief back one step. For example, ask yourself *why* being successful is a prerequisite for happiness. What rule is this belief based on? You might answer with "Success is necessary for any positive emotion."

4. Ask yourself whether you think this rule is true. Think about evidence for or against this rule. Do you know "unsuccessful" people who are happy, or "successful" people who are unhappy?

5. If you find the rule to be inaccurate, create a new one. If it is accurate, try to formulate it into a core, basic belief, like "Success is subjective" or "We all deserve happiness."

Following your beliefs is a good practice whether you want to get to sleep or not; it can lead you to empowering new insights.

stretch out your thoughts

Sometimes your thoughts can bounce around in your head like Ping-Pong balls, making it difficult to focus or relax. Use this technique to slow your thoughts by stretching them out:

1. With your eyes open, take 5 quick, deep breaths. Breathe in fully through your nose and blow the air out forcefully through your mouth.

2. Let your breath return to its normal rhythm and allow your eyes to gently close.

3. Settle in and start paying attention to your thoughts. Choose one of the thoughts that pops up and focus on it.

4. Instead of letting it pop in and out and moving your focus to a new thought that arises, let this one stretch out. For example, the thought might be "These pajama bottoms are comfortable." Instead of hurrying off to the next thought, let this one sit. Think about how comfortable these pajama bottoms are. Repeat the thought to yourself but at a much slower pace, letting it drag out. Activate your imagination and see the thought elongating in your mind.

5. When you feel you've covered that thought fully, let it go. When your next thought arises, repeat the same technique, stretching it out and settling into it.

This exercise helps your brain slip into a lower gear and move at a slower pace, preparing it for sleep.

engage your third eye

Whether you believe in any mystical powers of the third eye or not, there is something comforting about engaging your third eye. Try this technique to open up your third eye and find calm:

1. Close your eyes and bring your palms together in front of you with your fingers pointing up.

2. Breathe deeply, in through your nose and out through your mouth. On your third exhale, slowly bring your hands up to your forehead, keeping them pressed together gently.

3. As your thumbs brush the center of your forehead, allow your third eye to open. This should bring with it feelings of awareness, connectedness, and intention. With your third eye open, you are open to experiences, and you feel a sense of enlightenment and spiritual peace.

4. Hold your third eye open and allow all of these feelings to suffuse you. Feel them spreading to every corner of your body. Feel open and centered and aware.

5. Finally, use the path that these positive feelings are traveling to fill you with calm from the tips of your toes to the top of your head.

6. When you feel calm and at ease, allow your hands to fall by your sides and get into your favorite position for sleep.

You don't need to believe in the power of the third eye to reap the benefits of this exercise, so give yourself permission to give it a shot.

change your perspective

If you're feeling stuck in your head or your current perspective, try flipping the script by changing your *physical* perspective with a little change of scenery. Try these steps:

1. Before you get started, take a moment to simply sit where you are currently. Take a few breaths and think about where your mind goes, what you see, and how it feels to be in this exact spot in the room where you are sitting.

2. Now, look around you to find a new spot in the room. This spot should offer you a new physical perspective on the room you're in right now.

3. Move to your new spot, slowly and mindfully. Take a look around you. You're in the same room, but you'll notice that you have a completely different view of things. Notice what you can see now that you couldn't before. Note what looks different due to the angle or lighting differences.

4. Now, settle in and turn your attention to your thoughts. Has your mindset changed at all from this shift? Are you thinking about different topics or seeing things in a new light?

5. Use this phenomenon to your advantage. Head back to bed with the knowledge that you can shift your perspective by shifting your body, and let it shift into one of sleepiness.

Simple changes in your perception can have a big impact on your state of mind. Use this exercise to shift into a sleepier state.

gather up your gratitude

This exercise is part visualization and part thoughtful meditation, but it can lead to all relaxation. Here's how it works:

1. Find a cozy spot on your bed and get into a comfy seated position. Let your hands fall open, palms facing up.

2. Close your eyes and turn your attention to gratitude. What are you grateful for? What makes your life better and happier? What are you thankful for and appreciative of in your day-to-day life?

3. Visualize these things in front of you. See each of them in detail. For example, you might see an image of your partner or closest friend, an image of your office at work, or a graduation cap symbolizing all the things you've learned. Keep thinking of things to be grateful for, filling your vision with these blessings.

4. Now, take a deep breath in through your nose and imagine reaching out and gathering all of these things in your arms. Hug them close to you as you exhale.

5. Continue gathering up blessings and drawing them in until you can't think of anything else. Give them all a final mental squeeze, then release them on an exhale.

Sit in the state of contentment that all this gratitude left you with, and let it carry you to a serene slumber.

use soothing music

Music can have a profound impact on your mood and mindset, from energizing you to encouraging you to feel loving feelings. It can also be used to calm and soothe. This exercise incorporates soothing music to help you drift off to sleep. Here's how to do it:

1. **Find some calming music to put on. A quick web search should turn up lots of options.**

2. **Put the music on at a low volume, one that you have to sit still to hear. Then, get yourself into a comfortable sleeping position and close your eyes.**

3. **Begin to deepen your breath, letting your inhales and exhales elongate. Allow the music to fill your awareness.**

4. **Focus on the soothing sounds you are hearing. When thoughts pop up—as they inevitably will—let them gently pass by and turn your attention back to the music.**

5. **Follow the music in your mind, letting it fill you. Engage your ears like you never have before, pouring all of your attention and awareness into listening to the music.**

6. **With the music comes calmness, contentment, and relaxation. Allow these associated feelings to enter you with the music, spreading throughout your body and bringing a soothing sense of peace and sleepiness with them.**

Allowing yourself to feel the music in your mind and body might help you turn off your busy thoughts for the night.

follow your heartbeat

A heartbeat is one of the most relaxing and soothing sounds for humans. Given that most of us spent about nine comfortable, cocooned months hearing little else, it makes sense that we associate heartbeats with nurturing and peace. Use your own heartbeat to your advantage with this technique:

1. Turn off all sources of noise in your bedroom (e.g., silence your phone, turn off the fan, shut down the TV) and lie down on your bed. Choose your most comfortable side to sleep on and press that ear into your pillow. With one ear firmly blocked by your pillow and no other sounds, you should be able to pick up the faint beat of your heart. You can place a hand over your heart or on your wrist to help you find it.

2. Tune in to your heartbeat. Let your full awareness be taken over by the rhythmic beat of your heart. Remind yourself that you are listening to your own life; without a heart pumping blood through your veins, you wouldn't be here to listen for it. Think about how much work your heart is doing right now, sending precious oxygenated blood throughout your body.

3. Keep listening to your heartbeat, giving thanks for a functioning heart, and allowing it to soothe you. Sink into the calm, steady beat and match your mind to its rhythm.

Tuning in to the sound of your heart taps into the primal, powerful ability of the heartbeat to soothe and calm.

let your thoughts wash away

This meditation combines visualization with acceptance-focused meditation, leaving you calmer and more present. Here's what to do:

1. Sit upright on your bed and close your eyes.

2. In your mind's eye, create an image of yourself and your thoughts. See your thoughts popping up one at a time in your head. They might look like thought bubbles or strings of words typed out and jostling for space in your brain.

3. Watch as they grow larger in size, reflecting the attention you are paying to them. Now imagine them shrinking, and being replaced by other thoughts. See them arising, vying for attention, and disappearing, one after the other.

4. Now, visualize these thoughts moving at a slower pace and coexisting in your head.

5. Next, imagine a gentle stream of warm water flowing over your head. As you watch the water flowing over you, observe the thoughts slowly washing away. Continue washing them away until there is nothing left.

6. Sit in the stillness and appreciate the calm. Smile, lie back, and let yourself drift to dreamland.

This exercise evokes a gentle mental cleansing, which is likely to quiet your busy mind.

chapter four

emotion meditations

identify your emotions

To address emotional issues and get back to sleep, you need to first figure out what's actually going on with your emotions. Follow these steps to try a simple meditation to do just that:

1. With your eyes closed, think about what you're feeling right now. Find whatever that feeling is and sit with it. Allow it exist in you.

2. Try to come up with a label for it. Is it anger? Amusement? Confusion? Gratitude? Name it if you can.

3. If you have trouble identifying the feeling, try shifting your focus to your body for a bit. How does the emotion feel in your body? Is your chest tight or does your throat feel constricted? Then perhaps it's stress or sadness. Does your heart feel light and open? Maybe you're feeling compassion or contentment. Use your body's cues to figure out how your head is feeling.

4. Once you have an idea of what you're feeling, choose the label that makes the most sense. Try to be descriptive; instead of just "sad" you might feel "melancholy." Instead of feeling "happy" you might be feeling "joyous."

5. Sit with this feeling you've identified for a few moments, soaking in how it feels to experience this emotion.

It's impossible to accept and address your emotions if you don't know what they are. This exercise can help identify them.

trace your emotion
to the source

If you have a good idea of how you're feeling but don't understand why, that confusion might be keeping your brain too busy to sleep. Use this meditation to figure out where your feelings are coming from:

1. **Close your eyes and sit with your emotions for a moment. Figure out what emotion is primary right now. Make sure you have a good handle on the strongest emotion you're feeling.**

2. **Imagine a thread attached to the emotion you're feeling. You can see where the string is attached to the feeling, but you can't see where the rest of the string goes yet. Pick up the thread.**

3. **See yourself pulling on this thread, using one hand after the other, to discover more and more of its length. Stay present with your emotion while you do.**

4. **Follow it long enough, and you will start to see things pop up along this thread that fed into your emotion; for example, you might see a fight you recently had with your partner or an incident with a friend. Let these things come up, acknowledge them, and keep pulling the thread. Go all the way until you reach the source: the root of your current emotion.**

Sometimes all we need is to figure out where our feelings are coming from to let them go and let ourselves rest.

accept your emotions

Acceptance can help you let go of that which you don't need and fully relax, allowing you to drift off to a peaceful sleep. Follow this meditation to practice accepting your emotions:

1. First, identify and label your emotions (if you're not sure, the "Identify Your Emotions" meditation can help you do that). Understand what feelings you're working with.

2. Take a few moments to simply sit with one of your main feelings. Let it wash over you, sink into you, soak into your core. Get friendly with it.

3. Visualize the emotion. What does it look like? Does it look like a person? An animal? Just an abstract mix of shapes? However it looks, hold it in your mind's eye.

4. Face toward this visualization of your emotion and address it. Hold your hands up, palms open, and say, "I accept you." You can say it out loud if that helps. You can also imagine embracing the emotion.

5. Let the visualization melt away, accepting it as a part of your current experience.

At times, you may need to fight your demons in order to rest easy. At other times, you may just need to embrace and accept them as they are to allow yourself to relax.

see your emotions as colors

If you're a visual person, working with and through your emotions may be easier if you add a visual element. Emotions are abstract and can be hard to grasp, but assigning them a color and incorporating visualization can help you identify, accept, and understand your emotional self, making it easier to put your mind at ease and drift off to sleep. Here's how to try incorporating colors into your emotional work:

1. **Figure out how you're feeling in this moment. What emotion is at the forefront right now? What emotion seems to be the strongest? (The "Identify Your Emotions" meditation in this chapter can help if you're not sure.)**

2. **Identify and name the emotion you're feeling.**

3. **With your eyes closed, think about what color best suits your current emotion. Take a minute to find the color that fits.**

4. **Now, visualize your emotion with this color. It might be a pulsing ball of light in this color, a translucent ribbon like the northern lights, or even a canvas painted with this color. Sit with the feeling and let it grow and shift, and watch as your visualization grows and shifts along with it.**

5. **If you have multiple strong emotions, repeat this exercise for each emotion.**

Working *with* your emotions rather than *against* them is the best way to find peace and relaxation.

kindle some kindness

Do you chastise yourself when you can't get to sleep? Do you think, "What's wrong with me? Why can't I just turn off and go to sleep?" You might even mentally yell at yourself and your overactive mind, begging it to "Please, just shut up!" You probably already know that berating and criticizing yourself won't help you get back to sleep any quicker; what might help is cultivating and resting in kindness. Try this meditation to kindle some kindness:

1. **Think about the last time you experienced kindness.**

2. **Call to mind how it feels to be on the receiving end of kindness. How does it feel in your body, and in your head? What thoughts does it bring up? Does experiencing kindness have a color associated with it?**

3. **Grab onto that feeling and cultivate it. Expand on it and add to it, growing it into a bigger and bigger feeling.**

4. **Hold on tightly to that big, wonderful feeling of kindness. Let it soak in for a few moments.**

5. **Finally, send that experience of kindness to the critical voice in your head, gently shushing the voice and surrounding it with good feeling.**

Your first instinct may be to drive away critical and shaming voices, but this exercise will show you that drowning them with kindness is a much more effective method. With your nagging voice quieted, let yourself fall gently back to sleep.

neutralize frustration

When you're frustrated, it can be nearly impossible to get your mind calm enough for sleep. Frustration weighs heavily on you as you wait for sleep to come, but luckily the solution is simple: Find your frustration, acknowledge it, and neutralize it. Here's how to neutralize your frustration:

1. **In a comfortable position, close your eyes and take in a deep breath. Fill your lungs completely, then let all the air out in a rush through your mouth. Repeat this deep breath 5 times.**

2. **Think about what you're frustrated about.**

3. **Think about *why* this particular issue is causing you frustration. What is going differently than you'd like it to? Perhaps someone is not behaving in a way that you think they should. Figure out what rule or belief you hold that their behavior is violating.**

4. **Determine whether or not this rule or belief is a helpful one for you (hint: It's probably not).**

5. **If it isn't helpful, picture yourself letting go of this belief and replacing it with a newer, more realistic one.**

6. **Give yourself permission to rest.**

There are many ways to deal with frustration, and this is only one of those ways. Deep breathing, visualization, and body-focused meditations can also help you let go of your frustration and allow you to relax enough to get back to sleep.

remove doubt

Cozy in your bed but feeling doubt creep up in your head? Feeling doubt is a common reason people can't fall asleep. If you're using mental energy worrying and questioning things, you won't be able to shut down your mind and prepare for sleep. Instead of getting dragged down by doubt, try this meditation to remove it:

1. Sit comfortably with your eyes closed and a pen and piece of paper nearby. Think about what is keeping your brain busy with worry. What are you doubting? What are you concerned about?

2. Once you've identified the issue, ask yourself:

   - "Can I do anything about this right now?" If you can, do it. If you can't, write down your doubt and let it go.

   - "Is this coming from my authentic self or my fearful self?" If it's coming from your fearful self, give that fearful self a mental hug and soothe it back to a state of relaxation. If it's coming from your authentic self, write it down.

   - "Will this matter in a week? A year? Ten years?" If it won't matter, acknowledge the doubt and let it go. If it will, write it down.

This exercise is a quick way to figure out what's bothering you and, more importantly, what you can—or can't—do about it right now. As you will find, the answer is almost always to acknowledge it and let it go.

say goodbye to sadness

If you're unable to sleep because you are feeling a little sad, you may need to neutralize or set aside that sadness in order to rest. Try this meditation to alleviate some of your sadness so you can sleep:

1. Lying flat on your back with your eyes closed, picture sadness as a person. What does sadness look like? What is it wearing? See it in detail.

2. Sit with sadness for a few moments. Listen to what it has to say. Allow it to tell you what is causing the sadness and why it's here.

3. Comfort sadness if that feels natural. Perhaps place a hand on its arm or give it a warm hug.

4. Once it's done telling you why it's here, thank sadness for sitting with you. Tell sadness that you need to get back to sleep now, but you appreciate it for sharing its struggles with you.

5. Wave goodbye to sadness and watch it walk away. Relax fully into your bed.

Sadness is a sneaky emotion that can creep in when you're supposed to be at rest. It's not necessarily a bad thing—after all, sadness can be an effective cue that we're lacking something important or not living according to our values. But you don't need to dive into that when you're trying to get back to sleep; this emotion-focused visualization can help you acknowledge the sadness and let go of it.

find your peace

We are all in search of peace. It's not only a lovely feeling to experience; it also helps increase happiness, enhance well-being, and improve our ability to relax and rest. If you feel your midnight wakefulness could be helped with a sense of peace, give this meditation a try:

1. Close your eyes and think about the word "peace." What comes to mind when you consider the word? You might think of a Zen garden, a still pond, or perhaps a quiet grove of trees.

2. Whatever you associate with the word "peace," focus on it. Imagine it with as many specifics as you can. For example, if your association is a grove of trees, see it in detail using your senses: Imagine the color of the leaves, the texture of the bark, the color of sky peeking between the branches, the soft sound of birds chirping, and the smell of pine.

3. Transport yourself to this setting. Sit in the grass among these trees and breathe in the scent of the woods. Feel yourself sinking into the soft ground and hearing the gentle breeze as it rustles the leaves.

4. Allow a deep sense of peace to suffuse you. Sit with this sense of peace.

This meditation is almost guaranteed to get you into the gentle, relaxed state that precedes slipping back into sleep. If you're still alert, try sinking even deeper into the visualization and cataloging even more details.

create some happiness

When you're having trouble falling asleep, you might find yourself lacking in positive emotions; fueling some happiness can create the right context for sleep. Try this meditation to create a little happiness for yourself and allow your mind to relax:

1. **Rest in a seated position with your hands on your knees, palms up.**
2. **Take 5 deep, steady breaths, inhaling through your nose and exhaling through your mouth.**
3. **Zero in on the present moment, using your breath to stay grounded.**
4. **Turn all your attention to what you are currently hearing. List each thing you can hear.**
5. **Now, turn your attention to what you are feeling in your body. List each thing you can feel, like an itch or the pressure of your legs on the chair.**
6. **Adopt a gentle smile and allow the joy of being fully present to seep into you. Breathe in happiness for a few breaths, then lie back and relax into your bed.**

Happiness is the quintessential pleasant emotion, one that we spend a lot of time chasing; however, there's no need to chase it—you can find it by simply tuning in to the present moment. An added bonus of accessing positive emotions is their ability to calm and soothe, making it easier to shut off your brain and slip into sleep.

eliminate embarrassment

We all have moments when we think back to an embarrassing experience and find ourselves embarrassed all over again. This is totally normal, but it's certainly not conducive to sleep. Give this exercise a try to eliminate embarrassment and get back to a sleepy state:

1. **Bring to mind whatever event is bothering you. Run it through your mind so the experience feels fresh.**

2. **Now, think about yourself at that point in time. Who were you? What were you dealing with at the time? What were your big concerns or challenges at that point?**

3. **Tell yourself that you were doing the best you could with the resources you had at the time. Cultivate a little compassion for your embarrassed self.**

4. **Remind yourself that everyone has embarrassing moments, that we all make mistakes and do things we regret. Send out some of that compassion for everyone who has made an embarrassing move, including you.**

5. **Continue sending out compassion until you feel the embarrassment slipping away. Finish with a little hug for yourself if that feels right.**

Embarrassment is a natural and inevitable human emotion, but you don't need to hang on to it when it pops up. Use awareness and compassion to eliminate embarrassment and give yourself a break, allowing your mind to rest.

nurture self-compassion

Cultivating some extra self-compassion can be helpful when you're struggling to get back to sleep. Follow these instructions to nurture compassion for yourself:

1. **Lie in a comfortable position that feels nurturing for you. You might try curling up on your side or lying with your arms folded around your body.**

2. **Thinking about yourself, zoom out to see yourself from a third-person perspective. Try to see yourself as a stranger.**

3. **Knowing what you know about yourself, look closer at this person. Adopt a kindly perspective as you consider them.**

4. **Keeping in mind the challenges and struggles this person has faced, focus on all the good traits and characteristics. Think about how strong this person is to have survived to this point.**

5. **Tell this person how well they've done getting to where they are now.**

6. **Now, bring yourself back to the present, realizing that this person is you. Give yourself a big hug.**

Offering yourself compassion makes you happier, healthier, and more resilient. It's especially important to practice during times when you may be struggling to be kind to yourself, like when you're struggling to fall back to sleep.

let go of anger

There's nothing wrong with feeling anger. But when you're stewing instead of sleeping, try this meditation to let go of the anger that is not currently serving you:

1. Sit upright with a straight back and your hands resting on your knees or legs.

2. Find your anger and sit with it. Allow it to come up, along with whatever thoughts and feelings it brings with it.

3. Think about where your anger comes from. Identify the reason or explanation that makes sense to you.

4. Holding this reason in your head, clench all your muscles. Make your hands into fists and press them into your legs, flex your legs and tighten your shoulders, pulling them up to your neck. Pour all of your anger into your muscles, making your body tense and tight.

5. Hold your breath for a few seconds as you continue to flex everything.

6. In one swift action, release your breath in a big "whoosh" through your mouth, relax all your muscles, and mentally let go of this reason for being angry. Tell yourself that this is not serving you right now and allow it to float away.

Letting go of anger is a great way to relax and soften both the body and mind, making it easier to drift off to sleep.

soothe your fear

If fear is what's keeping you awake, use this meditation to identify and soothe your fears, allowing you to drift gently back to sleep. Here's how it works:

1. **Get into a comfortable seated position with your hands on your knees, palms up, and close your eyes.**

2. **Think about what is making you feel fearful. Is it something in your surroundings, something that's causing you immediate danger? (It's almost certainly not something that's causing you immediate danger. If so, get help right away!)**

3. **Identify the fear and vocalize it—either in your head or out loud. For example, you might say, "I'm afraid of messing up the presentation I need to give at work this week."**

4. **Now that you know what it is, picture this fear in your mind. What does it look like? Is it a person? An image of the situation you're afraid of? Just shapes or colors? Maybe it's more like a flickering light. Whatever it is, get a picture of it in your mind.**

5. **When you have a clear image of it, bring your hands up to your upper arms and give yourself a little squeeze. Tell the image, "Don't worry, I've got this."**

It might seem silly at first, but keep hugging yourself and repeating the phrase until the image gives off a little less fear than it did at first.

create a state of calm

Feeling calm is not only a pleasant experience; it's also really helpful for getting you back into a sleep-ready state if you've woken up in the middle of the night. Try this meditation to create a sense of calm for yourself. Follow these instructions:

1. Find a comfy spot on your bed and either lie down with your arms out at your sides, palms facing up, or sit upright with your hands on your knees, palms facing up.

2. As you get into position, focus your attention on your breathing. Is it short and shallow? Or maybe quick and uneven? To create a sense of calm, you'll need to shift your breathing to a slow and steady pace.

3. Close your eyes gently, then start to shift your breathing. Make your in-breaths a little bit longer, then make your out-breaths a little bit longer. Next, add a brief pause between each inhale and exhale.

4. Continue breathing in slow, steady breaths. Imagine yourself bringing in a sense of calm with each breath you take. With each inhale, you get a little calmer and more peaceful.

5. Take at least 10 breaths with this focus on creating calm, then let your breathing go back to normal and sit with your newfound sense of calm.

A sense of calm like this can travel throughout your body, bringing relaxation with it wherever it goes...like into dreamland.

save your excitement for later

If you have an event or occasion coming up that you're excited about, it can be pretty tough to get back to sleep. Excitement boosts your energy, enhances your mood, and prepares you for engagement—all good things, but not conducive to sleep. Try this meditation to take that excitement and store it away for later:

1. With your eyes closed, engage your imagination. First, visualize a container. It can be a box, a chest, a basket, a drawer, or anything else with a lid or top. Imagine this container in detail, from the shape, color, and size to the texture and any carvings or decorations it may have.

2. Shift your imagination to another subject: your excitement. Imagine a small version of yourself, giddy with excitement. This version of you is practically bouncing with anticipation and bursting with energy. See this tiny, adrenaline-filled version of yourself in detail.

3. Now, visualize yourself taking your tiny, excitement-filled self and putting them in the container. As you put them away, their excitement doesn't dim at all. You're simply storing all that energy and enthusiasm for later. And don't worry, they'll be fine in there for the night—and ready to pop out with gusto in the morning.

This meditation can be helpful for anyone, but it might be especially helpful for children who are too excited to sleep.

get rid of gloom

The more you try to avoid, deny, and/or push away your negative feelings, the more power you give them. Instead, use acceptance to acknowledge them and take some of their power away. Here's what to do:

1. Close your eyes and put your arms around yourself in a soft, soothing hug.

2. Acknowledge that you are feeling a little gloomy. This is not an admission of defeat but a statement of fact. You are, in fact, feeling a little down, and that's okay.

3. Tell yourself it's okay. Remind yourself that everyone has ups and downs, and it's totally fine to feel down. There is no rule that you must feel positive all the time.

4. Sit with your feelings for a moment, then rub your hands up and down your upper arms (or your legs, or your sides, or wherever feels comforting to you). Soothe those feelings instead of trying to rid yourself of them. Allow them to be, and offer them some comfort instead.

5. Continue giving yourself this loving embrace until the intensity of your negative feelings is a little lowered, then get into a cozy sleeping position and prepare for rest.

It's okay to feel gloomy, but this exercise can help you address your feelings and get back to sleep.

cultivate some grace

Grace is a specific emotional state that not only allows you to forgive and hold compassion for yourself and others; it is also a comforting, soothing state to be in. Use this calming meditation to cultivate some grace and soothe yourself back to sleep. Here's what to do:

1. Sit upright with your hands in your lap. Imagine there's a balloon tied to your head that is pulling your head up, making your back straight and your head lifted.

2. Turn your attention to yourself. How do you feel about yourself? We all have doubts and insecurities, but do you generally feel good about yourself? If so, take that good feeling and hold on to it. Feed it and allow it to grow, creating a sense of love and understanding for yourself.

3. If you're having trouble finding those feelings, call up some love and compassion for one of your loved ones. Build up those loving feelings, then shift them over to yourself.

4. Once you have these positive, compassionate feelings built up, extend them out toward all people.

5. With your eyes closed, take a deep breath. As you inhale, build up forgiveness and grace for all. As you exhale, release it and send it out to every human being, including yourself. Let yourself settle into a sleepy state.

Grace isn't something we usually think about on a daily basis, but creating some can be an effective tool for soothing ourselves to sleep.

surrender to relaxation

Sometimes, in order to take control and power through a difficult situation, we paradoxically need to let go. Use this meditation to practice surrendering:

1. Start in a seated position on your bed with your eyes closed. Make sure there is space behind you to lie down.

2. Take a few deep, steady breaths. Breathe in and out through your nose.

3. Think about what it is you're holding on to. What are you trying to control that you can't actually control? Maybe you're struggling to deal with another person's behavior, or maybe you're trying to plan for an uncertain situation.

4. Let go of whatever it is you're trying to control, whether it's another person, world events, or the weather. You can only control your own behavior, and trying to control anything else is an exercise in futility.

5. As you let go, physically surrender—lean all the way back onto your pillow and relax. Feel how good it is to let go.

6. Take another deep, calming breath and prepare for sleep.

"Surrender" is often thought of as a negative word, but that's not the only way to think about it. Sometimes the best way to get through a tough time is to give up control and just go with the flow.

develop an anxiety barrier

If you're already struggling with anxiety, the inability to fall asleep on schedule only adds to the burden. Instead of trying to remove all anxious feelings, try putting up an anxiety barrier. Here's how to do it:

1. With your eyes closed, bring up your feelings of anxiety.

2. Sit with these feelings, even though it might be a little uncomfortable. Pay attention to each thought that comes up. Imagine these thoughts are bouncing around you, knocking into you and causing you distress.

3. Now, visualize a bubble forming around you. This bubble is your anxiety barrier. See the shiny, transparent edge as it rises up on all sides. It might be clear, or it might be tinted with a color that you find soothing, but you can still see through it.

4. Watch as it slowly builds up and over your head, sealing you inside. It's warm and comfortable in this bubble, and now all the anxious thoughts are stuck outside. They're still bouncing against the barrier, trying to get in, but the bubble is impenetrable.

5. These anxious thoughts and feelings are still there, but now they're muted and distant. Get into your coziest sleeping posture and let sleep come naturally.

Visualizing this bubble protecting you for the night might just enable you to get some much-needed rest.

create contentment

Contentment is joy's less frenetic and more practical cousin. We all want to feel joy, but contentment is the calmer, longer-lasting, and more soothing emotion. If you can't sleep, try this meditation to build contentment:

1. **Choose your most comfortable position in this moment, whether it's sitting, lying, leaning, or even standing. Make sure you are at a cozy temperature; don't be afraid to grab another blanket or turn on a fan to get there.**

2. **With your eyes closed, put a gentle smile on your face. You might think that only positive feelings lead to a smile, but the process can work in reverse as well: A smile can lead to positive feelings.**

3. **Think about how wonderful it is to be here in this moment. You may not have everything you want, but you have a place to sleep, the clothing and/or bedding required to be comfortable, and yourself and your awareness.**

4. **Cultivate some gratitude for these very basic but very good things you have. Sit in this comfortable sense of gratitude and allow yourself to be content with where you are right now.**

We all want contentment—perhaps even more than happiness—but we sometimes get caught up in the idea that it should come to us. Instead, you can choose to rejoice that you can create that sense of contentment with just a little mental effort.

cry it out

If you're holding back tears right now—whether they're of frustration, anger, sadness, or simply feeling overwhelmed—letting them out can be the key to relaxing enough for sleep to take you. Try this meditation to let those tears flow:

1. First, make sure you have tissues handy, then get into a comfortable position on your bed.

2. Call to mind everything that's bothering you right now. Sit and stew in these feelings for a few moments.

3. Identify some of the thoughts that go along with these feelings. For example, if you're feeling frustrated, you might find an accompanying thought like "This situation will never get resolved."

4. Take a few minutes to just cry it out. Cry until you can't bring up another tear. Just let it all go.

5. Now, return to the thoughts you identified and come up with a more practical, less emotion-driven response. For example, you might respond with this: "Of course it will get resolved at some point; it's just hard to imagine that right now when I'm in the middle of it."

6. Dry your tears and remind yourself that it's good for you to just cry it out if you need to.

If you're just not a crier, that's okay—but give this meditation a try anyway. You might surprise yourself.

self-validate your emotions

When you're struggling, you might want someone to hear you, understand you, and empathize with you. If no one is there, all hope is not lost; you can validate yourself! Try this exercise to practice self-validation and to soothe your troubled mind back to sleep:

1. Start by taking an inventory of what's bothering you right now, either in your head or on paper. It might be one big thing, a bunch of little things, or a combination.

2. Look through your inventory and think about how each item is making you feel. For example, an item on your inventory might be, "My dad is ill." In that case, you might note, "It makes me feel anxious and concerned all the time."

3. For each item on your list, look at the item and its impact. Think about the connection between the two, and remind yourself that it's understandable to feel this way. Tell yourself that anyone in your shoes would feel the same way.

4. Continue until you finish your inventory. Close your eyes, take a deep breath, and let it all out in one big exhale while you tell yourself, "My feelings are understandable. It's okay to feel this way."

We often go to others when we need validation of our feelings, but that's tough to do when it's the middle of the night. It's also a great skill to be able to validate yourself.

connect with your heart

This meditation technique will help you reconnect with your heart, which allows you to find compassion for yourself and create a calm, relaxing energy. Here are the instructions:

1. Sit up on your bed with your legs crossed and your eyes open.

2. Stare straight ahead as you breathe in deeply through your nose and exhale through your mouth. After a few breaths, switch to breathing in and out through your nose.

3. Now, close your eyes and continue breathing slowly and steadily. Lift your left hand and place it gently over your heart. Settle into stillness and feel your heart beating underneath your palm.

4. Connect to your heart. Listen for the rhythm of the heartbeat. Tune in to that rhythm and begin to integrate it into your breath. For example, you might breathe in for 3 heartbeats, then breathe out for 3 heartbeats.

5. Feel the connection with your heart and sit with it. Revel in the sense of connectedness of mind and body.

6. Continue breathing steadily for a few moments, then let your hand drop to your side and finish with a big, deep breath in through the nose and out through the mouth. Lie back and allow sleep to find you.

Connecting your heartbeat and your breath will help you cultivate a feeling of deep, intimate self-love, creating a soothing state to help you relax.

engage your healing energy

You might not think of yourself as a healer, but we all have the potential to heal inside of us. In this meditation, you will engage your inner healing energy and allow it to gently rock you to sleep. Here's how to do it:

1. Start by sitting upright with a straight back and your hands resting on your knees. Close your eyes and focus your attention inward.

2. Think about what the idea of "healing" brings up for you. What images do you get? What thoughts or scenarios come up? Perhaps you think of a compassionate, caring nurse. Or maybe you think about loving, gentle hands.

3. Whatever healing thoughts or images come up, take a few moments to connect yourself to them. See yourself as a medical professional who is dedicated to the patient's care—the patient can also be you!

4. Allow yourself to embrace this healing energy and let it move through you. Feel yourself thrumming with energy.

5. Now, focus that energy to those parts of you that need healing the most. For example, send it to your heart and allow yourself to heal and mend and repair. Rest your hands on your heart during this time.

6. After a few minutes of healing, relax into rest.

Believe in your ability to heal and harness that power, and getting yourself to sleep will be just one of your many abilities.

burn up your negativity

If you are feeling pessimistic and you find comfort in a campfire, this meditation will help you rest while shedding negativity. Here's how:

1. In a comfortable meditation position, turn your attention to the negative feelings you have right now. Tune in to them.

2. What is your negativity saying? Take a few moments to see negative thoughts for what they are: evidence of a pessimistic perspective that your mind has adopted.

3. Remind yourself that this pessimism is one of many possible perspectives the mind could choose, and that you don't need to hold on to it if you don't want to.

4. Picture this negative perspective in your mind. You might see it as a swirling dark mass of energy or the proverbial half-empty glass. Try to see it as clearly as you can.

5. Now, imagine yourself setting fire to it.

6. See it burn as the flames dance around it, shifting from orange to yellow to red. Watch as it crackles and pops like a real fire. Carefully warm yourself in front of it.

7. As it burns, you can feel it taking the negative energy with it. Left in its place is a gentle optimism. Smile and embrace the cozy, comfortable new perspective.

Just as a phoenix rises from the ashes, allow this meditation to burn away all negativity and let you start fresh with a good night's sleep.

allow irritation to float away

Feeling irritation can make it tough to relax and get back to sleep. Try this exercise to release it and fall back to a peaceful sleep:

1. Sit upright with your legs crossed and your hands on your knees. Begin with 3 deep, intentional breaths, in through your nose and out through your mouth.

2. Close your eyes and let your breathing return to normal.

3. Now, tap in to your feelings of irritation. Think about what this irritation feels like to you. It might feel like a burning or twisting sensation inside of you.

4. Next, engage your imagination and picture the irritation. Does it look like a writhing mass of thorns? A bubbling pot of toxic stew? Create a strong mental image of it.

5. Expand your visualization to include a big body of water. The irritation is floating on a little raft in front of you.

6. Make a conscious decision to let go of the irritation. Give it a little push and watch as it slowly floats away.

7. Keep watching until it's so small you can barely see it, and then until it is gone completely. Take a deep breath and exhale, enjoying your newfound peace.

When you visualize physically letting go of things, you give your mind permission to let go and find a sense of peace.

apply serenity

This meditation exercise will help you create serenity and put it to use right now to help you feel calm, positive, and relaxed:

1. Get comfortable on your bed and check in with how you're feeling right now. If you're feeling a little tense or agitated, that's okay—just note how you feel.

2. Now, create some serenity for yourself. Flip your hands so your palms are up. Open up your chest by pulling your shoulders back and lifting your sternum. Curve your lips upward in a gentle smile.

3. Repeat the word "serenity" to yourself, either in your head or out loud. Think about what "serenity" means to you. Think of its synonyms and correlates, like "peace" and "tranquility." Say those words to yourself too.

4. Imagine yourself creating a tangible "serenity" product and bottling it up like lotion.

5. Finally, watch yourself open the bottle and apply its contents all over yourself. Smooth it over your arms and shoulders and rub it into your chest, letting it sink into your heart. Watch as serenity infuses you.

Try visualizing other positive emotions and experiences and "applying" them the same way.

change your emotional frequency

This meditation is a fun and easy way to get yourself in the right state of mind for sleep. Use a little visualization to change your emotional experience and soothe your busy or agitated brain. Here's how to do it:

1. First, get cozy on your bed and close your eyes. Take a few deep breaths to get centered and find stillness.

2. Tune in to your current emotional state. What are you feeling? Take a minute to simply identify what you're feeling right now.

3. Next, imagine a radio in front of you. It's an old-fashioned radio with a big silver knob you can turn in either direction to change the frequency, but this knob is labeled "emotional frequency."

4. Hit the power button, turning the radio on. You can see your current emotional state pop up on the radio. It says "stressed" or "bored" or whatever emotion you identified earlier.

5. Now, reach out and grab the knob, twisting it to the left or right. The displayed current emotional state rapidly changes to "content," and you feel a shift. Suddenly you actually *feel* content, peaceful, and at ease.

6. Twist the knob again, and you find "relaxed." Note that you can now feel a sense of relaxation in your body. Continue twisting the knob and finding different positive, soothing states.

7. Give the knob a final twist and let it land on "sleepy." Allow yourself to sink into sleepiness.

This emotion visualization is not only a good way to get to sleep; it also offers an opportunity for some comforting nostalgia if you had an old radio or boom box as a child.

create a nurturer

There are specific forms of therapy that involve creating images that you can connect to when you need something specific, like protection or wisdom. Follow these directions to create a nurturer who can lovingly soothe you to sleep:

1. **Close your eyes and bring to mind the concept of nurturing. What feels nurturing to you? What comes to mind may be a specific person you know, a person you don't know (like a generic "caring grandmother" archetype), or even an animal (like your childhood dog).**

2. **Whatever feels most nurturing and loving to you, focus on that. As an example, let's use a caring grandmother: Note what she looks like, what color and style her hair is, and the clothes she's wearing. Also note her kind facial expression, and imagine how it feels to get a hug from her. Be as detailed as you can.**

3. **Now, bring her to life. Tell her you're frustrated at not being able to sleep, and let her nurture and soothe you. You'll find that she says exactly what you need to hear to relax and rest.**

4. **Thank her and allow yourself to sink into sleep.**

Creating a nurturer won't just help you relax; it will also help you get through tough moments throughout your day-to-day life.

chapter five

visualization meditations

count the sleepy sheep

This meditation is a twist on the classic "count sheep to fall asleep" advice. You're still counting sheep, but instead of watching them jump over a fence, you're going to see them drifting off to dreamland. Follow these instructions to count sleepy sheep:

1. Visualize a peaceful meadow with rolling hills, green grass, and quaint wooden fences. See it in as much detail as possible, down to the nails in the fence and the flowers poking up through the blades of grass.

2. Imagine it is filled with fluffy white sheep, slowly milling about in small groups.

3. Choose a group and zoom in. As you zoom in, you see the sheep begin to lie down and rest their heads. Watch as they get comfortable in the soft, cozy grass.

4. When a sheep stops moving and closes its eyes, count that as 1. Look to the next sheep, and watch it do the same.

5. Continue counting until all the sheep in that group have fallen asleep.

6. Zoom out and pick another group, then repeat the steps until you have watched all the sheep float gently to sleep—or until you're asleep yourself.

Counting sheep can help, but counting *sleepy* sheep is a certified sleep hack.

float with the stars

Sometimes it helps to shift your perspective when you're struggling to get your mind to cooperate. One excellent way to do that is to think of the stars. Try this visualization to "zoom out" to play with the stars:

1. **Lie flat on your back with your arms at your sides and your legs stretched out long. Close your eyes.**

2. **Picture the night sky: an impossibly black backdrop with thousands upon thousands of tiny pinpricks of light. See the many galaxies, clouds of stars, and stardust strewn across the sky.**

3. **Watch as your body lifts up to join the sky. See it rise gently all the way up to float with the stars.**

4. **Look around you with wonder. Take some artistic liberty and play with your surroundings; you might see the planets orbiting around you, catch shooting stars blasting through space, or even witness stars dancing with one another.**

5. **Allow this fantastical world to delight and soothe you. If things are moving, slow them down to a gentle crawl, then stop the motion altogether.**

6. **Feel your body floating with ease as you view the brilliant, calm, wonderful scene around you.**

Getting into your body can help you drift to sleep, but so can putting some distance between you and your current worries; visualizing yourself floating with the stars can do just that.

let sleep wash over you

In this visualization, you will use your imagination to see and feel sleep as a fluid thing, allowing it to wash over you and gently rock you to sleep. Here's how it works:

1. Lie in your bed in a comfortable position, preferably on your back, with your eyes closed.

2. Now, think of "sleep" as a body of water with a gentle tide lapping at the shore—perhaps a lake, a pond, or a lagoon. Visualize this calm, soothing place as the water rises and falls along the shoreline.

3. Imagine yourself lying by the edge of this body of water, with your feet toward the water. You are comfortable, warm, and safe.

4. Watch as the tide rises and the water gradually moves toward you. It reaches your feet, gently lapping at your heels.

5. The tide softly recedes, then comes back, the water reaching up to your ankles this time. Watch as it recedes once more, then gently rushes up to your calves.

6. Continue watching as the tide gently reaches higher and higher up your body. As the water reaches your neck, remember that the water is sleep in this visualization. It reaches your mouth and nose, and you realize that you

can still breathe, but you are breathing in a sense of calm and peace with each inhale. If having water near your head makes you anxious, simply imagine the water stopping at your chest.

7. As the water covers your entire body, allow it to gently rock you to sleep.

This meditation harnesses the soothing power of water to get you quickly back into a sleepy state of mind.

try a tree cocoon

If you're someone who feels soothed by nature (and are not worried by the idea of small spaces), this meditation will be a soothing breath of fresh air. Follow these instructions to make yourself a tree cocoon:

1. Lie on your side with your knees drawn up as far as feels comfortable for you (i.e., the fetal position).

2. With your eyes closed, imagine that you are lying in the branches of a beautiful, vibrantly green tree. You can see yourself and the tree from a third-person point of view, and you are in awe at how lovely the tree looks and how peaceful you look in its branches.

3. As you look at yourself in this tree, you notice that the tree's leaves and vines are slowly shifting. They are moving toward you, softly and with love.

4. Watch as they gather around you, weaving into a soft place to rest. They join together, entwined around your body, creating a soft, soothing cocoon of nature.

5. The cocoon is solid underneath you, holding you in safety. But you can see through the vines and leaves above you to get a glimpse of the upper branches and the night sky.

6. Feel the warmth and love as the tree pulses to gently soothe you to sleep.

If you like to cocoon yourself in your blankets, this is a great visualization for inducing a sense of sleepiness.

weave a grass blanket

Grass often looks more comfortable than it feels in reality, but with this exercise, you can create the reality you want. Use this visual meditation to create a soft, cozy blanket out of grass:

1. With your eyes closed, imagine you are in a field of gently swaying grass. The grass is a stunning shade of green against a beautiful blue sky.

2. Walk through the field, running your hands over the grass. Notice how soft and smooth the grass feels.

3. Find a nice spot to lie down. Get comfortable and look at the grass around you.

4. Watch as the grass begins to bend and sway toward you. It moves slowly and carefully, reaching out for other stalks of grass as it goes. They move over and under and around one another, weaving themselves into a soft, cozy blanket. See the grass folding itself into this blanket just for you.

5. As the grass completes its weaving process, it slowly lowers the blanket down onto you. You can feel the warmth and gentle weight as it lands.

6. Close your eyes and shift into your favorite sleep position, pulling the grass blanket around you.

The combination of the beautiful scenery and the soothing feel of a soft blanket will lull your mind into a relaxed state, ready for sleep.

float down a river

If you have ever floated on a calm river before, you know it can be an incredibly relaxing experience. This visualization will place you on a gently flowing river and allow you to float your way to a peaceful sleep. Here's how to do it:

1. Lie in a comfortable position (this works better than sitting for this particular visualization).

2. In your mind's eye, bring up a vision of a slow-moving river in a beautiful, vibrant setting. Imagine the banks of the river teeming with green life. See the crystal clear water reflecting the soft blue of the sky and occasionally glinting with the light of the sun.

3. Now, imagine yourself floating atop this river. Your body is naturally buoyant, lying just on top of the water. Feel the warm, comfortable temperature of the water on your back.

4. Look up and see the blue sky filled with soft, fluffy white clouds. Feel the gentle waves as they rock up and down your body, carrying you slowly down this beautiful river.

5. As you float in this visualization, allow your eyes to softly close. Relax your entire body and allow the water to move you downstream as you drift closer and closer to sleep.

Water is a great addition to any visualization meant to create calm. Its fluid state makes it seem gentle and soothing. Use a slowly moving source of water to help lull you to sleep.

create a white light

This is a simple and generic visualization meditation that you can use anytime you need a boost of good feelings. Use it now to soothe your busy mind and create the right context for sleep. Here's how to do it:

1. Imagine yourself in a dark, warm, and comfortable place. You are safe, but you feel something is missing. You look around yourself, but you see nothing but darkness.

2. As you strain your eyes to see something, a tiny, faint white light appears. You can barely see it; it's nothing but a spark—but it's something other than darkness.

3. You can feel a soft mental glow coming off it. The light is emitting waves of positivity, calmness, and contentedness.

4. Realize that you willed this white light into existence; your wish has called it into being, and you imbued it with the good feelings it brings.

5. Since you created it, you can control it. Set your mind to expanding this white light. Watch as it grows bigger and brighter, bathing you in its soft, soothing light.

6. Continue growing it bigger and bigger until it not only reaches you but it surrounds and engulfs you. You are completely contained within the soft, warm, calming light. Close your eyes and allow yourself to relax fully into it.

It might seem counterintuitive to invoke light, but this visualization uses light to soothe you instead of to energize you.

lie in a field

Nature can have a soothing, calming presence that allows you to shut off your busy brain and relax into sleep. Use this visual meditation of lying in a field to harness the gentle power of nature:

1. As you lie comfortably in your bed, allow your imagination to roam. Travel through places you've been, places you've seen pictures of, and places you've dreamed about, keeping an eye out for the right field.

2. Once you've found it, you'll know. It will fill you with a sense of peace and a calmness and serenity that instantly puts you at ease. See this field in as much detail as you can, from the color of the sky to the shape of the stalks of grass to the gentle movement in the field caused by the breeze.

3. Find a cozy-looking spot in the field and lie down, feeling cushioned by the soft earth beneath you. The ground has been warmed by the sun, and that warmth now seeps into you.

4. Look up above you at a patch of the bluest sky you've ever seen, peppered by fluffy white clouds and framed by the softly swaying green grass. Sink into this moment, in this place, and surrender to serenity.

Judging by how often they are used in movies and TV to represent relaxation and peace, fields have a special place in our hearts. Create your own peaceful field to find your way to sleep.

visualize a loved one

If you're feeling agitated or anxious, calling to mind someone whom you associate with love and caring can be just the right medicine to soothe your mind. Focusing on a dearly loved person in your life will help you feel calm and collected. Here's how to do it:

1. Think of someone you feel very loving toward. It could be a parent, a child, a significant other, or a very dear friend. It should be someone who matches your love for them, making you feel safe, special, and cared for.

2. Imagine them standing before you. See this person in as much detail as you can, from the style of their hair and the flecks of color in their eyes to what shoes they're wearing. Get a clear image of them.

3. Now, see yourself standing in front of them in your mind's eye, facing toward them. See yourself in detail as well.

4. Imagine that you are smiling at each other, and all the love and care you have for each other is in those smiles. Feel the connection between you, and feel the love flowing in each direction.

5. Soak in the love they send you, and send just as much in return. Rest in that love and surrender to it.

You'll find after this meditation that you somehow have *more* love in your heart, even though you sent and received an equal amount of love.

see the sounds

Sometimes sounds can distract our mind from the important task of falling asleep; however, that's not always the case. This meditation combines sounds and visualization to soothe you back to sleep:

1. Once you're in a comfortable position, start by closing your eyes and breathing in deeply through your nose, then exhaling completely through your mouth.

2. Bring your attention to the sounds you hear around you. Observe and note each one. For example, you may hear your fan blowing air, the wind rustling through the trees, a dog barking down the street, or birds chirping up above.

3. Now, pick one sound and focus on it. Use your imagination to visualize where the sound is coming from. For example, you might pick the wind rustling through the trees. See it in detail: the shape and color of the leaves, the branches they are attached to, and the wind gently whistling by as it flutters the leaves.

4. Repeat this exercise for each sound you hear until you have a vision of all of them.

5. "See" all of the sounds, creating a peaceful picture of everything you hear. Allow that peace to seep into you.

Connecting your senses with meditations like these can create a deeper, broader sense of peace than using one sense alone.

visualize yourself sleeping

It may sound silly at first, but you can put visualization to good use in the middle of the night by seeing yourself sleeping. Visualizing yourself in a peaceful slumber will essentially "trick" your mind into believing it can sleep. Use this meditation to try it for yourself:

1. Sit upright with your back straight and your eyes closed.

2. Engage your imagination and see yourself all tucked into your bed, cozy and comfy. See this image in detail, from your position and the clothes you're wearing to the color of your sheets and the headboard behind you.

3. Once you have this image in mind, allow this imaginary you to breathe. Watch as you take the deep, slow breaths of sleep. See your eyelids flutter and your fingers twitch as you sink deeper into sleep.

4. Let the calmness of your sleeping self transfer from the version of yourself in the visualization to yourself in the present moment.

5. Continue cultivating this sense of peace as you lie back in your bed and get into the sleeping position you visualized. Breathe in and out steadily and allow sleep to find you.

Note the pleasure with which you get into a comfy position after seeing yourself sleeping so peacefully in it. Connecting your imagination with your outer reality can help you find balance and tranquility.

take a mental walk

If you can't get back to sleep and you're feeling stuck in your current environment, go somewhere else in your mind. Use this visualization to envision a peaceful, calming environment that will put you at ease. Follow these instructions to try this visualization meditation:

1. With your eyes closed, picture yourself in a peaceful, natural setting. You might choose a lake, the woods, or by the ocean. Whatever you choose, it should be a setting that feels most calming to you.

2. Once you have this setting firmly in mind, find a path and begin your mental walk.

3. In your imagination, you have no need to watch where you step, so take advantage of this benefit of visualization and look around as you go. Look left, look right, and look above, seeing all the beauty that surrounds you.

4. Stroll slowly through your preferred landscape, stopping to look closely at anything you find extra-pleasing or peaceful. When you pause, take a moment to breathe in deeply, noting the sounds and smells of your surroundings as well as the sights.

5. Let the peaceful environment relax your mind and body, and sink into your bed, ready for sleep.

Slow, peaceful strolls are great for the body *and* the mind, whether they're real or imaginary.

look out over a canyon

If you've ever visited the Grand Canyon, you know how awe-inducingly beautiful it is. It creates a sense of wonder and connection with nature that can put the mind at ease and the body at rest. Follow these steps to invoke the sense of wonder and peace that a natural setting like a deep canyon can provide:

1. **Close your eyes and picture yourself on the edge of a vast, deep canyon. The rim reaches as far as you can see to your left and right, but you can see the other edge a great distance away.**

2. **Look down and see how deep the canyon goes. Notice how the color of the cliff shifts and changes depending on the height.**

3. **Look out and see the varied landscape of red earth, white rock, green trees, and gray stone. Scan across the canyon and see the beautiful shifts in color and texture.**

4. **Think about how long it took to carve this canyon out of the ground, and all the tons of rushing water that flowed through it.**

5. **Breathe in gratitude for the beautiful surroundings and allow the all-encompassing peace of nature to suffuse you.**

Many natural sights can create a sense of wonder, joy, and contentment, but a vast canyon may be the most peace-inducing of all.

design your dream vacation

Design your dream scenario and allow the relaxation and carefree feeling of vacation to lull you back to sleep. Here's how:

1. Ask yourself what place sounds most relaxing to you. Is it the beach? A rainforest bungalow? Perhaps a cozy cottage on a snow-covered mountain? Pick the place that makes you feel most at home and at ease.

2. Imagine you have two weeks of vacation to use and just the right amount of money to plan a trip to this beautiful, relaxing spot. What kind of trip would you book?

3. Think of at least a few fun activities you would engage in during this trip, like skiing, hiking, or scuba diving.

4. Think of a few relaxing activities you would incorporate on your trip, like getting a massage, taking guilt-free naps during the day, or reading a good book in a cozy spot.

5. Finally, think about the lovely people you would spend this trip with, whether that's family, friends, or strangers.

6. Live out this trip in your mind, hitting all the highlights. Imagine how relaxed you would be on this trip.

7. Breathe in deeply, exhale, and allow sleep to take you— perhaps to enjoy another visit to your dream location.

Treating yourself—whether it's in reality or in your mind—is a great way to feel calmer and more relaxed.

relax in a hammock

Hammocks cradle you in a way that few things can, allowing you to rock back and forth as you sink deeper into comfort. Follow these steps:

1. Lie back with a pillow under your head and another pillow or a rolled-up blanket under your knees. This will create a similar feeling to being in a hammock.

2. Close your eyes and place your hands on your stomach.

3. Envision a soft, cozy hammock strung up between two tall, leafy trees. It's swaying slowly in a gentle breeze, dappled by hints of sun filtering through the branches above it.

4. See yourself walking over to the hammock and climbing in. Feel the smooth texture of the hammock under your hands. Feel the hammock hold your weight as you sit down and lean back all the way.

5. Allow the breeze to gently rock you from side to side in the hammock, making your body sway in a comforting rhythm. You may want to rock gently back and forth in your bed to feel the sway in your own body.

6. Close your eyes in your visualization as well and feel the warm sun against your face. Let the rocking motion lull you to sleep.

Visualizing yourself in a hammock is almost as good as the real thing—try it and see if sleep soon creeps up on you.

recline in a cloud

Have you ever looked up at a fluffy white cloud and thought, "That looks cozy!" If so, this is the visualization for you:

1. Lie back in a comfortable position. Get under the covers or a blanket for maximum coziness, then close your eyes.

2. Picture a crisp blue sky above you. It's a beautiful, sunny day and the sky is a vibrant, cheerful blue. As you watch the sky, you can see small, fluffy clouds begin to drift into your view.

3. Pick the coziest, most pleasant-looking cloud and zoom in on it. Imagine yourself floating up to meet it.

4. When you get to the cloud, see yourself stepping onto it and being supported. Feel the bouncy, cushioned spring of the cloud as you walk on it. Find the coziest-looking spot and lie down.

5. In your reclined position, get comfy and look around you. See the beautiful blue sky and the soft white clouds and the sun shining. Feel its warmth on your face as you relax into your cloud.

6. Take a few deep, slow breaths. Feel your cloud gently rising and falling with your breath, mimicking the inhale and exhale as it gently rocks you to sleep.

Give yourself a soft place to rest with this visualization.

stroll through the jungle

The jungle might not sound like a safe place to relax, but jungle sounds are a popular choice on sound machines. Know that you're in a safe, secure place while you enjoy this meditation:

1. In a cozy position on your bed, take a few steady, soothing breaths to get centered. Close your eyes and engage your mind's eye.

2. Imagine a tropical jungle. What does it look like? What does it sound like? What does it *feel* like?

3. See the jungle in detail. Visualize the bright colors of the jungle's many flowers and vines. See the rough, detailed bark on the trees. Watch as shiny green and brown leaves fall from the sky and drift down to the ground.

4. Walk through this jungle, putting one foot in front of the other and taking it all in. Hear the songs sung by jungle birds and the playful calls of the monkeys in the trees. Notice how the sounds shift around you as you walk.

5. Feel the gentle condensation on your skin and the warm breeze as it ruffles your hair. Touch the big, broad leaf of a nearby plant and note the texture.

6. Find a soft, comfortable spot on the warm jungle floor and sit down, allowing your body to relax.

When you put yourself in a calming three-dimensional space, you invite your body and mind to sync and relax.

play in a waterfall

The low roar of the falling water provides a comfortable white noise that allows you to disengage your busy thoughts and calm your mind. Use this waterfall visualization to bring a sense of serenity to your mind:

1. After you get into a comfortable position on your bed, take a few soothing, slow breaths to relax your body. Close your eyes and open your imagination.

2. Think of a waterfall. What comes up? Is there a specific waterfall or a sort of default waterfall that comes to mind? Get the image of this waterfall firmly in mind.

3. Once you can easily see the waterfall, see yourself getting up from your bed and standing in front of the waterfall. Watch as you slowly stroll over to the waterfall. Notice how the sound of the waterfall gets louder as you approach.

4. When you reach the waterfall, hold out your hand—palm up—and feel the water as it cascades over your hand. Notice that the water feels surprisingly warm, almost as if it's from a warm bath and not a spring-fed stream.

5. Look up and see the water falling down toward you. Take a step into the waterfall and feel it cascading over your head and shoulders. Let the warm, rushing water wash away your tension and stress, leaving only serenity in their place.

Water is a great element to add to relaxation-focused meditations, whether it's still or flowing.

vacuum out the energy

This whimsical meditation will help you relax and induce a sense of calmness in your body as you prepare for sleep. Here's how to do it:

1. Lie down on your back and close your eyes.

2. Imagine that you have a very fancy vacuum that you can attach to your head. This vacuum doesn't suck up air like normal vacuums do; it sucks up energy. Picture how this vacuum would look.

3. Now, attach this vacuum to the top of your head and turn it on. It doesn't make a loud sound, just a quiet hum.

4. As you breathe in, you can see the energy in your body gathering in your center, right around your ribs. Feel the energy gathering there from all four limbs.

5. As you breathe out, watch that gathered energy being sucked up into the vacuum attached to your head. Feel the energy rushing out of your body as it travels up your body and into the hose.

6. Continue breathing and feeling the energy gathering and leaving your body until your body is all out of energy.

7. Notice the difference in how you feel now versus when you began. Feel the quiet, calm, tired sensation now that all the energy has been sucked out of your body.

This silly-seeming visualization might make you laugh, but it will also soothe your busy mind.

explore a snowflake

Snowflakes are not only intricately detailed and beautiful; they can also lead your mind to relaxation through their association (e.g., holidays, sitting by the fire in a warm, cozy cabin). Here's how:

1. Sit on your bed and get under the covers to get cozy and warm. Close your eyes.

2. Imagine you are somewhere beautiful and wild out in nature. As you stand in this beautiful, wild place, looking around, you notice that it is beginning to snow.

3. Watch as the flakes slowly, almost lazily, drift to the ground. Find one that's about at eye level and press a metaphorical pause button, freezing it in midair.

4. Walk toward this snowflake. It becomes bigger and bigger in your mind's eye, until it's so big that it's all you can see.

5. Visualize the snowflake getting so big that you can step onto it and walk around on it.

6. Stop walking and look around, doing a slow 360-degree spin. Everywhere you look is the shiny frosty glint of pure white snow.

7. Bring your awareness back to your body, feeling the warm comfort of your bed.

After you finish this meditation, cultivate gratitude for your ability to appreciate such a beautiful sight while still being warm and cozy.

relax on the beach

One of the most popular choices for a relaxing vacation is the beach, but the real beach comes with coarse sand, noisy seagulls, and the sounds of other people. Use visualization to get the best parts of the beach and avoid the annoyances. Here's how:

1. Get cozy on your bed and lie back, then close your eyes.

2. Breathe in steadily through your nose and out through your mouth for 3 breaths.

3. Relax into the bed and engage your imagination. Visualize a beautiful beach with soft, white sand and crystal clear water. The sky is a deep blue with a few small white clouds, and the sun is shining down on you.

4. Stand on the beach with your toes in the sand. Notice the soft, luxurious feeling of it underneath your feet. Feel the warmth of the sun as it gently kisses your skin.

5. Lie down on the beach, letting the warm sand support you completely. Stretch out and settle in.

6. Allow the sounds of the beach to fill your mind. Hear the dull roar of the ocean as its waves crash down, and the soft "shhh" sound as the water recedes.

7. Let the warmth and peace of the beach infuse you. Allow it to fill you with a sense of calm.

The beach is the ultimate place for relaxation, especially when it's a perfect dream beach.

weather the storm

Some people find storms awe-inspiring, others relaxing, and still others think they are downright scary. If you like the sound of rain falling on the window, give this stormy visualization a try. Here's how to do it:

1. Lie back in a comfortable position. Take a few deep, centering breaths as you relax into the bed beneath you. On an exhale, allow your eyes to gently close.

2. Imagine you are sitting in a comfy seat by a window. Outside, you can see a cloudy gray sky, and it's darkening even more as you watch.

3. Rain starts gently falling. You can see the drops landing on the ground outside. You look up and see the raindrops framed against the dark sky. The speed of the raindrops picks up, and now it's raining heavily.

4. You wrap a blanket around yourself, grateful to be inside. As you sit comfortably, watching the rain fall, you see the first crack of lightning race across the sky.

5. The intensity of the storm is increasing and the wind begins to howl, but you feel no fear. You know you are safe and sound inside your warm house with a cozy blanket.

6. Watch the rain continue to fall for a few more minutes, then let go of the visualization and sink into your bed.

This visualization meditation will show you that if you can weather a storm, you can certainly soothe yourself back to sleep.

visualize the coziest bed

Your bed can look pretty inviting when you're tired and ready to hit the hay. Use this visualization to give an even bigger boost to your sleepiness. Here's how to do it:

1. Get comfortable in your bed first, then allow your eyes to gently close.

2. Imagine walking into a warm, softly lit bedroom. In this bedroom is the coziest, most comfortable bed you've ever seen. There are soft, cloudlike blankets on top of it and cozy pillows at the head of the bed. See the bed in detail.

3. See yourself walking toward the bed. The closer you get, the comfier it looks.

4. Sit down and feel it supporting you. It's the exact density and softness that you prefer.

5. Now, lie down and stretch out on the bed, pulling the covers over you. Feel the super-soft sheets, the incredibly comfortable mattress beneath you, and the perfectly warm covers on top of you. Settle in and enjoy the feelings of comfort for a few moments.

6. In your cozy, comfortable state, bring your awareness back to the present and the bed you're in.

When you finish this meditation, give thanks to your bed for being as cozy and supportive as it is.

sit in grandma's kitchen

If you had a warm, loving grandmother who loved to cook or bake for you, you probably have a great, comforting image in your head just from reading the title of this meditation. If not, that's okay—you'll create a nice, cozy space in this visualization exercise. Follow these steps:

1. **When you're seated comfortably on your bed, close your eyes and turn your attention to your mind's eye.**

2. **Imagine you are in your grandmother's kitchen (or think of another beloved family member or create one that you'd love to have). You're sitting at the kitchen table as she bustles around, baking bread or cookies.**

3. **Feel the chair underneath you, supporting you. Reach out and feel the smooth wood of the kitchen table under your hands. Feel the soft cushion underneath you.**

4. **Keep your eyes closed in your visualization so you can focus completely on the smells. Sniff the air for the aroma of what she's baking. Take a deep, delicious breath in through your nose and release it through your mouth.**

5. **Immerse yourself fully in this familiar world and sink a little deeper into your bed, relaxed and ready for sleep.**

Using all of your senses to place yourself in a cozy, comfortable place will give your mind leave to drift off to sleep.

watch the northern lights

The northern lights are a beautiful, natural display of how solar winds can affect the earth's atmosphere. If you've never seen them, take a moment to do a quick web search for them so you have an idea of what they look like. When you're ready, follow these instructions:

1. Lie flat on your back with your arms by your sides and your legs straight out. Close your eyes.

2. Take a very deep breath, the deepest you've taken all day, then release it through your mouth with a sigh.

3. Now, imagine you are up north, somewhere that's snowy and dark and remote. You're bundled up so you're not cold, but you can see your breath against the dark night sky.

4. As you look up at the sky, you notice a ribbon of light appear overhead. It's bright green and rippling gently through the sky. Suddenly, it turns blue. Now purple. Now pink.

5. Several more ribbons appear, slowly weaving through the sky and changing colors before your eyes. It fills you with a sense of wonder and comfort. You smile and continue enjoying the light show above you.

6. After a few minutes, the colors begin to fade. The lights dim, and all around you is a cozy, comfortable darkness.

7. Roll onto your favorite side and let yourself drift off to sleep.

Shimmery, shifting lights will gently drop you into a sleepier state of mind in this exercise.

enjoy a crackling fire

Staring into a fire is just plain mesmerizing. If you're struggling to get back to sleep, visualize a campfire to soothe your busy brain into a state of relaxation. Here's how to do it:

1. Sit upright on your bed with your legs crossed and your hands on your legs or knees.

2. Begin breathing gently in and out through your nose. As you find a sense of calm through slow, steady breaths, envision yourself sitting in front of a crackling fire.

3. Visualize yourself sitting in a comfortable chair and staring into the fire. The flames dance and throw shadows on the ground. The flames are a beautiful bright blue at the source, turning to orange and then yellow at the top.

4. As you watch the flames, you can hear the crackles as the fire devours the wood. Occasionally you hear a loud pop from the sap boiling inside the logs.

5. Close your eyes in the visualization and breathe deeply, inhaling the smell of a comfy campfire. Listen for the crickets, or any other pleasant nature sounds.

6. Feel the warmth of the fire on your hands and face. Allow that warmth to suffuse you, bringing a sense of serenity.

If you're a fan of campfires, this meditation should do the trick to get you back to sleep in no time.

watch the sun set

Sunsets are magical, not only for their inherent beauty and the sense of wonder they can provoke but also in their ability to signal to our brains that it's time for rest. If you missed the sunset tonight, don't worry—you can create your own. Here's how:

1. Prop yourself up in your bed with a pillow or two behind you and lean back, relaxing into the pillows. Pull your knees up and rest your arms on them.

2. Sit comfortably and allow your mind to rest for a minute, then close your eyes and begin to deepen your breath.

3. Use your imagination to whisk yourself away to somewhere you find beautiful and enticing, and where you have a good view of the sky. This might be a rooftop, on the beach, or even on top of a mountain.

4. Look out at the sky in front of you. See the bright blue of the sky above slowly shifting and fading to a reddish orange color with the sun sinking toward the horizon.

5. As you watch, the sky gently begins to darken. The sky goes from blue to purple, then orange and pink, and finally becomes a deep royal blue as the sun sinks all the way below the horizon and you drift off to a peaceful sleep.

When you are done, feel a sense of gratitude for being able to enjoy something as beautiful as a sunset.

visualize a ball of relaxation

In this visualization exercise, you'll replace the proverbial stress ball with a relaxation ball. Here's how:

1. In a seated position on your bed, sit upright with a straight back and your legs crossed, making space around you.

2. Close your eyes and put your hands together in front of you. Touch them together, palm to palm.

3. Now, imagine that you can gather up all the stress and tension inside of you and put it into your palms. Imagine the tension coming out in a dark, pulsing light between your palms. Move your hands farther apart as it grows, making room for it. Watch as it grows, taking all the tension out of your body.

4. When all the tension is out of your body and into your hands, take a moment to look at it. See how big it is, and notice how much tension you must have had.

5. Next, focus your attention on the ball. Send positive thoughts and energy toward it, and watch as it turns from black to gray, then gray to white.

6. See it turn all the way to white, and note how it feels to hold it now; instead of tension and negativity, you're holding a comforting ball of relaxation.

We often associate balls with sports and play, but this ball brings only associations of peace and calm.

row on a moonlit pond

This visualization pairs the natural serenity of water with the soothing glow of moonlight for a relaxing, calming exercise that will get you ready for sleep. Follow these steps to try it:

1. Sit on your bed with your legs out in front of you, like you're sitting in a rowboat. If that feels uncomfortable, you can bring your knees up to find a comfy posture.

2. With your eyes closed, let your mind wander to a calm, serene pond. The pond is quiet and the surface is still. The grass near the shore is tall and waving gently in the breeze. Watch as the last splashes of sunlight fade from the sky as the sun disappears behind the horizon.

3. Now, imagine yourself in a rowboat on this pond. You push off from shore and pick up the oars, slowly paddling out toward the middle of the pond.

4. As you row, the moon rises, creating a path of moonlight on the water. You can hear crickets chirping on the shore and an owl hooting occasionally from the trees.

5. Stop for a moment and put your oars down. Simply sit and float, taking in the moonlight, the water, and the sounds. Breathe deeply, allow yourself to relax into the moment, and appreciate this beautiful snapshot of nature.

Moonlight is a powerful tool in your imagination tool kit, injecting some peace and serenity into your experience.

find your sleepy place

If someone is stressed or irritable, they're often told to go to their "happy place." Happy places are great, but sleepy places can also be useful. Use this exercise to create one for yourself:

1. Lie on your bed in your favorite sleeping position. Make sure you're in comfy clothes and that you're warm and cozy in your bed.

2. Now, think about what your best sleeping conditions are. Consider the lighting in the room (pitch black versus a nightlight), the temperature (a little chilly or on the warmer side), the mattress (soft versus firm), the covers (a big, thick comforter or a thin, light quilt), and the sounds (silence versus a sound machine).

3. Think about the conditions under which you get your best sleep and all these different aspects of a "sleepy place." Make a decision about each of them, building your ideal sleepy place one piece at a time.

4. Once you have your sleepy place designed, close your eyes and transport yourself there. Settle in deeply and enjoy being in this comfortable, customized space. Allow sleepiness to take over and your body to relax completely.

Once you have your sleepy place set up, you can come back to it every time you need a little rest and relaxation. Eventually, your mind will associate calm and sleepiness with this place, and take you to your desired state automatically.